Praise for the *Intelligent Patient Guide* series

*The guide to breast cancer walks you through each step of
your diagnosis, treatment and prognosis...with explanations
that are easily understood. It brought everything together,
making it so clear.*
— J. McIntosh, Patient

*A guide not only to breast cancer but to breast health
and early detection of disease, the* Intelligent Patient Guide
to Breast Cancer *should be part of* every *woman's
personal library.*
— Cheryl Edwards MA
High School Teacher

*One of the best explanations of breast cancer risk I've seen
in print...dispells the 'panic' of the 'I in 9' statistics...
It's lovely to see in print many of the teachings we use
on a daily basis.*
— Barbara Warren RN
Director of Nursing,
Manitoba Cancer Treatment and Research Foundation

*As a patient advocate and breast cancer survivor, I lend
and use my copy of the* Intelligent Patient Guide *often.
The book helps equip patients to better understand the need
to take charge in the design of their own survival.*
— B. Cameron

*It was so informative. I felt so secure knowing what was
going to happen with every step.*
— D. Powell, Patient

Intelligent Patient Guide To

Breast Cancer

Other books in the *Intelligent Patient Guide*
series include:

Prostate Cancer
by S. Larry Goldenberg MD
ISBN 0-9696125-3-2

Colon and Rectal Cancer
by Michael E. Pezim MD
ISBN 0-9696125-0-8

Intelligent Patient Guide To

Breast Cancer

*All you need to know to take
an active part in your treatment*

Ivo Olivotto MD
Karen Gelmon MD
Urve Kuusk MD

edited by
Carol Glegg BSc

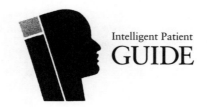

Intelligent Patient
GUIDE

Second edition, Vancouver, 1998

Distributed by **Gordon Soules Book Publishers Ltd.**
1359 Ambleside Lane, West Vancouver, BC Canada V7T 2Y9
PMB 620, 1916 Pike Place #12, Seattle, WA 98101-1097, US
604-922-6588 Fax: 604-688-5442 E-mail: books@gordonsoules.com
Web site: http://www.gordonsoules.com

While the authors have made every effort to ensure that the material contained herein is accurate at time of publication, new discoveries or changes in treatment practices may ultimately invalidate some of the information presented here.

Intelligent Patient Guide Ltd.
Vancouver, British Columbia
Canada
email: info@ipguide.com
Fax: 604 876 9334

Canadian Cataloguing in Publication Data
Olivotto, Ivo, 1956-
  The Intelligent Patient Guide to Breast Cancer:
  All you need to know to take an active part in your treatment

  (Intelligent Patient Guide)
  2nd edition.
  Includes index.
  ISBN 0-9696125-4-0

  1. Breast—Cancer—Popular works. I. Gelmon, Karen, 1953-
  II. Kuusk, Urve, 1950 - III. Glegg, Carol, IV. Title. V. Title:
  Breast Cancer. VI. Series.
RC280.B8055 1998   616.99'499   C98-900167-9

Typeset in Sabon by Résolutique Globale, Montreal
Cover design by Chris Dahl, Art & Design, West Vancouver
Printed in Canada

This book is dedicated to the thousands of women who have lived and are living with breast cancer and who, through their stories and their strength, have taught us so much.

Part of the proceeds from the sale of this book will go towards programs of Breast Cancer information, support and research.

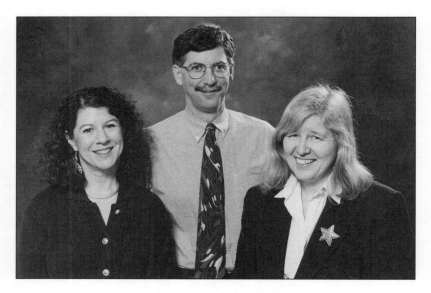

Authors (from left to right):
Karen Gelmon MD, Ivo Olivotto MD, and Urve Kuusk MD

Authors
Ivo Olivotto, MD, FRCPC
Chair, Breast Tumor Group,
British Columbia Cancer Agency;
Clinical Professor,
Division of Radiation Oncology,
University of British Columbia

Karen Gelmon, MD, FRCPC
Head, Section of Investigational New Drugs,
British Columbia Cancer Agency;
Clinical Associate Professor,
Division of Medical Oncology,
University of British Columbia

Urve Kuusk, MD, FRCSC
Clinical Assistant Professor,
Division of General Surgery,
University of British Columbia

Editor
Carol Glegg, BSc

Illustrator
Jane Rowlands, BSc (Art as Applied to Medicine)

Coordinator
Nicola Sutton, BA, MBA

Contributor
Maria Issa, PhD

Contributing Authors

Carolyn Baker, RN
Clinical Nurse Specialist
Vancouver Hospital & Health Sciences Centre

Judith Caldwell
President, Canadian Breast Cancer Foundation
British Columbia Chapter

Patricia Clugston MD, FACS, FRCS
Head, Section of Reconstructive Breast Surgery
Division of Plastic Surgery, University of British Columbia

Paula Gordon MD, FRCPC
Clinical Associate Professor, Department of Radiology
University of British Columbia

Susan Harris PT, PhD
Professor, School of Physiotherapy
University of British Columbia

Shirley Hobenshield, RDN
Registered Dietitian-Nutritionist
British Columbia Cancer Agency

Maria Hugi MD, FACEP
Emergency Room Physician and
Co-Chair, Treasure Chests Support Group
Vancouver, BC

Charmaine Kim-Sing MD, FRCPC
Medical Leader, Hereditary Cancer Program
British Columbia Cancer Agency
and University of British Columbia

Cheri Kutynec, MSc, RDN
Registered Dietician-Nutritionist
British Columbia Cancer Agency

Lis Smith, CCH
Clinical Hypnotherapist
Division of Patient and Family Counselling
British Columbia Cancer Agency

Richard Warren, MD, FRCSC
Head, Division of Plastic Surgery
University of British Columbia

Why read this book?

AFTER YOUR DOCTOR SAYS the words 'breast cancer' you may be in a state of shock. Despite this, you will be expected to make a series of major decisions, often in a hurry. 'Should I have a mastectomy? Should I have radiation? Chemotherapy? Tamoxifen?' The choices seem so complicated. Women often end up wondering, 'Should I just leave the decisions up to my doctors and do whatever they suggest?'

We believe not. Time and again we have seen that the patient who takes an active part in making the decisions that affect the course of her treatment is better able to cope than the patient who relegates all control to her doctors. While we are not advocating that you make choices independently of the recommendations of your doctor, we encourage you to become one of the decision-makers.

We wrote this book in 1994 to provide you with the information you will need to fulfill this role. It is gratifying that many women have found it useful. However, progress is being made and, as a result, we have extensively updated many sections and added two new chapters.

It is important to note that the statistics we have quoted about risks and prognosis refer to general or 'average' situations. Special additional circumstances may modify your individual risk and need to be discussed with your doctor.

We hope this book can help you move through the fear, to a place of hope and strength and the promise of life ahead — in spite of breast cancer.

Ivo Olivotto MD
Karen Gelmon MD
Urve Kuusk MD

Table of Contents

CONTINUED

PART ONE | **Breast cancer: What is it and how is it detected?**

SECTION ONE

The Normal Breast

CHAPTER ONE

Breast anatomy and function

THE BREAST IS MUCH MORE EXTENSIVE than most people realize.
(Figure 1). Breast tissue can be found as high as the collar bone
(clavicle), and extends from almost the middle of the chest over
the breast bone (sternum) to the armpit (axilla).

What's in the breast?

The breast is made up of milk glands, tubes (ducts) that carry
the milk to the nipple, and fat.

The milk is produced in hundreds of thousands of tiny glands
within the breast called lobules (Figure 2). The lobules are
drained by small ducts that collect the milk into larger glands
that look like tiny bunches of grapes. From here, big ducts carry
the milk to the nipple. The nipple surface contains about 20
duct openings, each draining a different part of the breast. All
the milk glands are cushioned by fat. The normal 'lumps' that
you feel in your breast every day are a combination of the milk
glands, fat, and other fibrous tissues.

The proportion of milk glands, ducts and fat in the breast
changes as you get older. During puberty, and as the breast
develops it consists mainly of ducts. However, in a 20-year-old

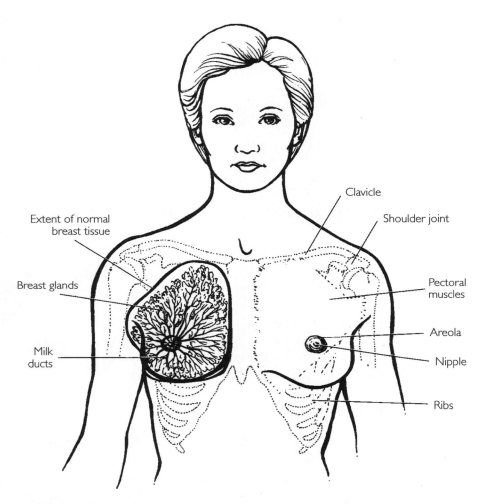

Clavicle

Shoulder joint

Extent of normal
breast tissue

Breast glands

Pectoral
muscles

Milk
ducts

Areola

Nipple

Ribs

Figure 1: Extent of normal breast tissue and important underlying structures.

woman most of the breast is made up of milk glands. During pregnancy and breastfeeding (lactation) the glandular content of the breast increases dramatically as the breast becomes prepared to produce milk.

The fat content increases as you age, especially after menopause. In an elderly woman almost all of the breast is fatty tissue. However, hormones taken after menopause maintain the glandular tissue and delay the normal fatty replacement.

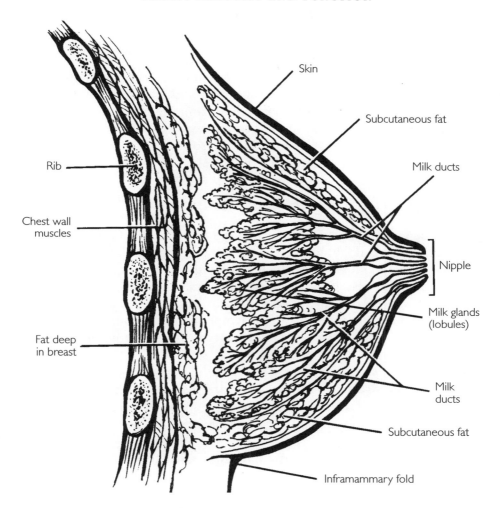

Figure 2: A cross-sectional view of the breast showing the internal appearance of the breast and its relationship to the chest wall.

Ligaments help hold the breast in place

Throughout the breast there are many supporting ligaments, like very thick, strong elastic bands, that connect onto the breast bone or muscles under the breast. With age, these ligaments tend to stretch and the normal breast begins to sag.

Muscles around the breast

A large, fan-shaped muscle lies beneath most of the breast. This is the *pectoralis major* muscle which is responsible for some of the movements of the shoulder and arm. You can feel this muscle as a firm ridge extending from the outside edge of the breast toward the armpit if you tense your arm and 'push in' with your hand on your hip. The *pectoralis minor* muscle is smaller and is not readily felt.

Lymph nodes: where infection fighting occurs

The purpose of the lymphatic system is to fight off infections in the body. Like blood vessels, there are tiny lymph vessels in every organ and tissue of the body. Fluid which normally leaks out of blood vessels to bathe the body tissues is collected by the lymph vessels and carried to groups of lymph nodes located at various places in the body. In the lymph nodes infections are 'filtered out' and destroyed. The 'treated' fluid then enters the blood stream.

Figure 3 shows the location of the main groups of lymph nodes that drain the breast. They are just above the armpit, above the collarbone, and along the sternum (the internal mammary lymph nodes). You have between 30 and 50 lymph nodes in the armpit.

Lymph nodes are of particular importance in breast cancer. Breast cancer cells sometimes enter the lymphatic vessels that drain the breast and may be carried to the lymph nodes where they settle and grow. The single most important factor in determining the future behavior of a breast cancer is if any cancer cells are found to be living and growing within the lymph nodes at the time of diagnosis (see Chapter 15).

Sensation and the nerves around the breast

Many nerves pass through the breast to the skin and to the nipple. In addition, the intercostal-brachial nerves come from the area between the ribs, through the armpit (axilla) and reach

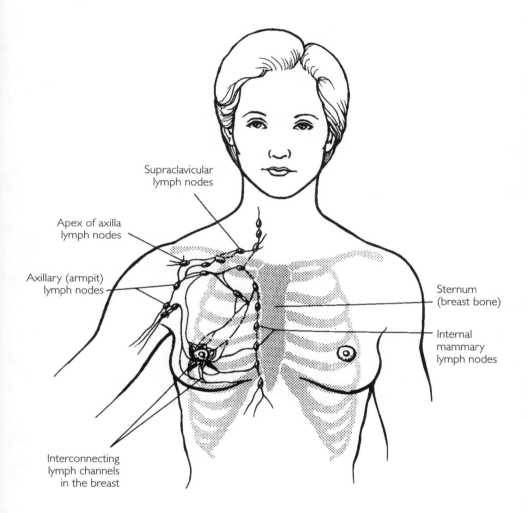

Supraclavicular
lymph nodes

Apex of axilla
lymph nodes

Axillary (armpit)
lymph nodes

Sternum
(breast bone)

Internal
mammary
lymph nodes

Interconnecting
lymph channels
in the breast

Figure 3: System of lymph nodes that drain the breast.

to the underside or back of the upper arm. These nerves are
often stretched or cut during surgery in the armpit which leads
to an unpleasant tingling, burning, numb or 'thick' sensation on
the back or underside of the upper arm. This may fade partly or
completely over several months after surgery, but if the nerves
have been cut, the numbness is permanent.

SECTION TWO

What Is Breast Cancer?

CHAPTER TWO

What is cancer?

To UNDERSTAND WHAT CANCER IS, it is important to first understand how the body's cells normally work.

How does the body grow and maintain itself?

The body is made up of tiny cells, for example, skin cells, muscle cells, heart cells, nerve cells and bone cells. When a baby grows the number of cells increases very quickly. A cell becomes a bit larger, then divides into two 'daughter' cells (Figure 4). After a period of time each of these cells divides again, and so on.

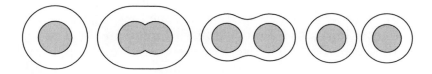

Figure 4: Normal cell division. A cell grows a bit larger and then divides into two cells.

Once a child grows to adulthood the size of the body no longer increases. However, our bodies go through a lot of wear and tear, both inside and outside. 'Upkeep' means that worn-out cells constantly need to be replaced, so cell division still takes place, but more slowly. An obvious 'outside' change is the tiny bits of dead skin flaking off as the skin constantly renews itself.

Although our bodies' cells continue to divide to replace worn-out cells, this happens in a very ordered, systematic way. The reason is that each cell carries genetic 'instructions' that regulate how fast the cell should divide and 'grow' and when the cell should die. A balance between cells growing and dying keeps our bodies functioning normally.

When cell growth goes out of control

Benign growths

Sometimes a cell starts to grow without regard for the normal balance between cell growth and death, and a small, harmless lump of cells will form. These harmless growths are referred to as 'benign.' A benign growth can occur in any part of the body, including the breast, skin or intestine.

Malignant growths

In other cases a cell may grow and divide with complete disregard for the needs and limitations of the body. They have the potential to grow into large masses or spread to other areas of the body. Cells that have this aggressive behavior are called 'malignant.' More commonly, a mass of such cells is called a 'cancer.' When clumps of these cells spread to other parts of the body they are termed 'metastases.' A cancer that continues to grow can eventually overwhelm and destroy the part of the body or particular organ where it is located.

Cancer cells also have the ability to stimulate the development of blood vessels to increase their own blood supply and enhance their growth. Sometimes, however, a cancer's wild growth rate backfires. The cancer may grow so rapidly that it can't get enough oxygen and nutrients from the blood vessels. When this happens a part of the cancer may suddenly die. This death of a group of cells within a cancer is known as 'necrosis.'

Cancer cells have the ability to spread

In addition to controlled growth, most normal cells remain in the area where they belong and don't spread to other parts of the body. Cancer cells disregard this principle and may spread through the body (metastasize) in several ways (Figure 5). These include direct invasion and destruction of the organ of origin, or spread through the lymphatic system and/or blood stream to distant organs such as the lungs, liver and bones.

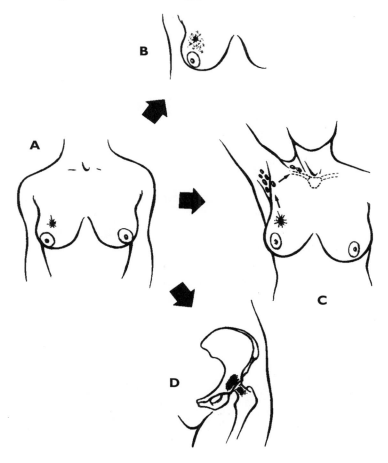

Figure 5: Mechanisms of spread of a breast cancer. A cancer (A) grows and spreads by direct local invasion (B) of the breast itself or (C) through the lymphatic system to lymph nodes or (D) through the blood stream to distant organs such as the bones, lungs, liver or brain.

When a cancer spreads it retains the properties of the original cancer. This means that a breast cancer that spreads to the bones is still a breast cancer. Under the microscope it looks different from a cancer that started in the bones, and it responds to treatment like a breast cancer, not a bone cancer.

The original cancer in the breast is called the 'primary' cancer. A cancer that has spread to another site is called a 'secondary' or 'metastatic' cancer.

Cancer cells can trick the immune system

The immune system consists of a group of cells called 'white blood cells,' specialized to recognize and destroy 'foreign' material in the body such as bacteria, viruses and unfamiliar or abnormal cells. Cancer cells somehow manage to slip through this detection system without triggering the immune system to start fighting, either at the primary cancer site, in the blood vessels, or at the site of distant spread.

Breast cancer does not develop overnight

It can take years of cells dividing before a normal cell becomes a cancerous cell. The cell first undergoes very small changes in which it becomes slightly abnormal or 'atypical' as seen under a microscope. It may also begin to divide, grow more quickly and accumulate in excessive numbers (hyperplasia). Then, over the years the cells continue to change, become more abnormal-looking and finally cancerous (Figure 6).

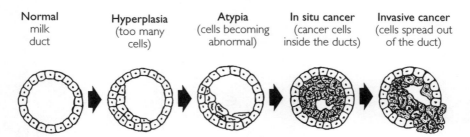

| Normal
milk
duct | Hyperplasia
(too many
cells) | Atypia
(cells becoming
abnormal) | In situ cancer
(cancer cells
inside the ducts) | Invasive cancer
(cells spread out
of the duct) |

Figure 6: Breast cancer does not develop overnight. Gradually the cells become more abnormal-looking or atypical (see text). Eventually, the cells are recognized as being sufficiently abnormal to be called cancer cells that are initially inside the milk ducts (in situ cancer), and later become invasive breast cancer cells.

Initially the cancer cells are confined within the milk ducts (in situ cancers), but with time the cells develop the ability to invade out of the ducts and into the blood and lymphatic system (an invasive cancer).

Unfortunately, it is not possible to detect one or a few abnormal or cancer cells. At present, technology is only capable of detecting a small lump or mass of cancer cells that has already started to grow. By the time a cancer can be detected as a lump, it may have been growing slowly for anywhere from two to eight years.

CHAPTER THREE

How common is breast cancer?

BREAST CANCER IS THE MOST COMMON type of cancer in women. In 1998 there will be over 19,000 new cases diagnosed and 6,000 deaths from breast cancer in Canada and approximately ten times that number in the USA. Breast cancer accounts for 4% of all deaths of women in North America each year and the loss of thousands of productive years of life.

'One in nine' is misleading

One often hears that 'one in ten' or 'one in nine' (lately even 'one in eight') women will get breast cancer. The trouble with these figures is that they are misleading because they don't tell the whole story. The figure 'one in nine,' for example, refers to the chance that a woman will develop breast cancer *if she lives to the age of 90*. A crucial point to realize, however, is that the risk of breast cancer increases with increasing age. Women over 70, for example, are at least four times more likely to get breast cancer than women who are under 40 years old. Not only that, but the majority of women die before the age of 90, so they don't reach the oldest age group where the high risk of breast cancer accumulates and pushes the overall lifetime risk up to 'one in nine.' For most women, therefore, the risk of getting breast cancer is much lower than one in nine.

Recent changes in the incidence of breast cancer

Since the 1940s there has been a slow but steady increase in the number of new cases of breast cancer diagnosed each year in North America. (The number of new cases diagnosed each year per 100,000 women is called the 'incidence.') This increase has been attributed to changes in nutrition (more calories) and changes in the reproductive patterns of women in North America. Today, women start menstruating several years earlier, delay having babies and have many fewer children. All these factors tend to increase exposure of the maturing breast to estrogens and have been linked to the higher rates of breast cancer.

In addition, a sudden increase in the incidence of breast cancer (more than 1% per year) has been seen since the mid-1980s. Much of this recent increase has been attributed to the increased use of screening mammography that has occurred since then. This is because screening mammography can detect some cancers two to five years before they would reach the size where a lump can be felt by the woman or her doctor. However, once the entire population undergoes mammographic screening at least once, then this sudden 'wave' of earlier detected cancers will become the new standard, and the incidence rates should drop.

You can estimate your own risk

Rather than considering a lifetime risk to age 90, a more useful question is: 'What is my risk, given my current age?'

Table 1 shows the average risk each year of developing breast cancer for typical North American women at specific ages. Using Table 1, based on her current age, the 'average' woman can estimate her risk of developing breast cancer over the next year. The risk over the next decade is 10 times the annual risk. For example, if you are 42, your annual risk is slightly higher than that of the 40-year-old listed in Table 1, say 1/1,000 per year. Over the next decade your risk would be 10 × 1/1,000 = 1/100 or approximately 1%. This risk is much easier to live with than one in nine.

Table 1	**Annual (not lifetime) risk of developing breast cancer**
At age	Risk
30 years	1 in 6,000 per year
40 years	1 in 1,200 per year
50 years	1 in 550 per year
60 years	1 in 400 per year
70 years	1 in 300 per year
80 years	1 in 250 per year

Table 2 shows not the annual risk, but the lifetime risk up to certain ages. As you can see from Table 2, even a woman who is 75 years old does not yet have a 'one in nine' chance of developing breast cancer. More specific, individualized risk estimates can be determined by considering additional factors that are associated with a higher risk of developing breast cancer, and then multiplying the 'average' risk at a certain age by the risk factor. Chapter 4 discusses some of the causes of breast cancer and ranks them according to their importance.

Table 2	**Chance of developing breast cancer by a given age**
Age	Lifetime risk
by 25 years	less than 1 in 1,000
by 50 years	1 in 63
by 75 years	1 in 15
by 90 years	1 in 9

CHAPTER FOUR

What causes breast cancer?

Why me?

'WHY DID I GET BREAST CANCER?' This is a question that doctors can almost never answer with any accuracy. However, it is not your 'fault' or 'punishment' for something you did or did not do and is not something you subconsciously 'needed.' Breast cancer is not something to be ashamed of.

There has been a lot of controversy over the years about the possible causes of breast cancer: diet, hormones, genetic make-up, or substances in the environment. Today we realize that there is no single factor that causes breast cancer, but that it is a combination of things, some more important than others.

What is a risk factor?

A 'risk factor' refers to something that increases your chances of getting a disease, in this case, breast cancer. A strong risk factor greatly increases the chances, while a weak risk factor just slightly increases your chances. For example, in the case of lung cancer, smoking is a very strong risk factor. In other words, someone who smokes is far more likely to get lung cancer than someone who doesn't.

With breast cancer there are several known risk factors, ranging from strong to weak (see Table 3).

A 'strong' risk factor is defined as something that increases the chance of getting breast cancer by more than four times (compared to someone without this risk factor). 'Moderate' means an increase of two to four times the risk, and 'weak' means less than two times the risk.

Strong risk factors

Increasing age is a strong risk factor for developing breast cancer. Women who are 50 years old have double the risk of women who are 40, and the risk doubles again by the age of 70 years (see Table 1, p. 20). For three-quarters of women who get breast cancer, getting older is the only identifiable risk factor. The remaining 25% of women with breast cancer have a combination of other risk factors.

Previous history of breast cancer

Most women who get one breast cancer do not get another. However, every year about one in every 200 women with a first breast cancer will develop another cancer in the opposite breast. Women with the lobular type of breast cancer (see Chapter 15) have a higher yearly chance, about one in every 100, of getting cancer in the opposite breast. Since there is no proven way to prevent these cancers other than by removing the entire opposite breast, it is important to keep the second breast under surveillance with regular self-examinations and examinations conducted by your physician, and an annual mammogram (breast x-ray).

Family history of breast cancer

A family history of breast cancer in a close relative such as your mother, sister, or daughter contributes to your risk. However, breast cancer in a more distant relative such as an aunt or grandmother has little or no impact on your risk. A history of breast cancer in a premenopausal close relative, breast cancer in more than one close relative, or cancer in both breasts of a close relative confers a four to six times higher risk of devel-

Table 3	**Risk factors associated with the development of breast cancer**	
Strong (Risk greater than 4× normal)	Moderate (Risk greater than 2-4× normal)	Weak (Risk greater than 1-2× normal)
Female sex	Over 30 years old at birth of first child	First menses before the age of 12 years
Advancing age		Menopause after the age of 54 years
Previous cancer in one breast (especially lobular carcinoma)	Past breast biopsy: any sign of cell abnormality or hyperplasia	Family history of breast cancer: older, postmenopausal
Family history of breast cancer: premenopausal or in both breasts	Postmenopausal obesity	Prolonged hormone use (more than 15 years)
Past breast biopsy showing severely abnormal cells and hyperplasia	Diet (possibly)	Moderate to heavy alcohol consumption
		Ethnic origin

oping breast cancer compared to a woman of the same age who does not have relatives with breast cancer.

There are rare families in which three or more generations have several relatives with breast cancer. In some of these families the disease may be passed on by a specific genetic mutation. For example, families with the BRCA1 gene inherit a tendency to develop both breast and ovarian cancer. Women who inherit such a mutation have a lifetime risk of developing breast cancer as high as 79%. Many of these families are characterized by breast cancer developing before the age of 50. The disease may appear five to ten years earlier with each generation (see Chapter 42).

Moderate risk factors

Later pregnancy

The delivery of a first child before the age of 20 causes hormonal changes in the breast tissue which provide modest protection against breast cancer. Delaying the first child until after the age of 30 or delivering no children increases the risk two to four times. Breastfeeding may decrease the chance of getting breast cancer by a small amount.

Previous breast biopsy showing abnormal cells or excessive accumulation of cells (hyperplasia)

As described in Chapter 1, a normal cell becomes a cancer cell through a series of changes in which the cells begin to divide and accumulate in excessive numbers (hyperplasia), become abnormal (atypical) and finally develop into cancer cells. If hyperplasia is seen in tissue removed during a breast biopsy, especially with atypical cells, the woman has a two to four times greater chance of developing breast cancer compared to a woman without these changes. If there is severe atypia and hyperplasia, especially in a woman who also has a family history of breast cancer, an eight-fold increased risk can be expected.

Weak risk factors

Generally, women who use oral contraceptives do not increase their risk of breast cancer. Some studies suggest that there is a modestly higher risk among women who, when they were young, took the older, high-dose estrogen type pill for many years (more than seven to ten years continuously). Modern oral contraceptive pills have a lower estrogen content, so that with 10 to 15 years of use they can be considered to cause no appreciable increase in the risk of developing breast cancer.

The onset of menstrual periods before the age of 12 years and cessation of menstruation after the age of 52 years weakly increase the risk of breast cancer.

Postmenopausal estrogen

The risk associated with postmenopausal estrogen use ('hormone replacement therapy') is more controversial. Overall, women who have at some point used estrogen alone (Premarin® and others) or estrogen in combination with progesterone (Provera® and others) do not have a higher chance of developing breast cancer as compared with women who have never used these medications. However, women who have taken post-menopausal hormones for longer than 15 years have an approximately 1.5-fold increased risk compared to the risk among non-users. This modestly higher breast cancer risk following long-term hormone use has to be considered in context with the potentially beneficial effects of these medications, including, among other things, a lower risk of bone fractures, fewer heart attacks and strokes, and relief of hot flashes, vaginal dryness and mood swings which may accompany menopause.

Diet and body weight

There has been extensive research into the role of diet in the formation of breast cancer. Some authorities believe that up to 30% of breast cancers may be attributable to dietary influences.

Studies of populations which move from an area associated with low breast cancer risk (e.g. Japan) to an area of high risk (e.g. North America) show that within one to two generations the migrant population adopts the risk level of the new country. This is thought to be due to changes of diet and life style which the children and grandchildren of the immigrants adopt.

It is not clear which dietary factors are important. The principal culprit thought to be associated with breast cancer is dietary fat, but this is still not proven. Furthermore, it is not known which type of dietary fat may be the culprit: saturated or unsaturated, fat of vegetable or animal origin, or whether the effect is simply related to overeating.

Moderate to heavy alcohol consumption (more than three drinks or six glasses of wine per week) has been associated with a weak increase in the risk of developing breast cancer. However, it remains reasonable to have an occasional drink or glass of wine.

Obesity during the postmenopausal years has been associated with a small increase in breast cancer risk. Interestingly, being markedly underweight in the premenopausal years also increases the risk, while premenopausal obesity does not.

Environmental factors

Radiation from x-rays is a common concern. Even at low doses, the use of x-rays in younger women (less than 20 years old) has been associated with an increased risk of breast cancer. However, the usual dose of radiation from a mammogram (x-ray of the breast) is very small. Most authorities estimate that the risk of inducing a breast cancer is extremely small compared to the benefit that a mammogram may find breast cancer when it is smaller and treatment is more effective (see Chapter 6). Also, routine mammograms tend to be used in women older than 40 who are more resistant to the effects of radiation than younger women.

Chemical carcinogens are everywhere in our environment, but no specific chemical or substance has been identified as specifically causing a greater number of breast cancers. Although recently there has been concern about organochlorines found in pesticides, so far there is no association confirmed between the use of pesticides and incidence of breast cancer.

Smoking does not appear to either increase or decrease the risk of developing breast cancer.

Race: little if any effect on risk

Historically, in the USA, blacks have had a lower incidence of breast cancer than whites, but unfortunately the survival rate for blacks is lower than the survival rate for whites. This has been attributed to differences in access to medical care. In Canada, the age-adjusted risk among First Nations women seems to be lower than that among caucasians.

Since ethnic groups who migrate to North America from areas of low risk (e.g. Japan and Southeast Asia) adopt the higher risk of the 'average' woman in North America within one to two generations, this strongly suggests that the influences of race, ethnic background and genetics have little, if any role compared to diet, life style or other environmental factors.

CHAPTER FIVE

Prevention – Is it possible?

Risk factors we cannot change

IT IS FRUSTRATING that the major known risk factors for developing breast cancer cannot be changed, such as female sex, advancing age, family or previous personal history of breast cancer and the age at which menstrual periods begin (see Chapter 4). Getting pregnant at a very young age may have a weak protective effect but there are many reasons why delaying pregnancy may be more important.

Risk and health factors that we can change

Life style factors

Life style changes have been shown to reduce the chance of developing heart attacks, strokes and some cancers. Stopping smoking definitely reduces the chance of getting lung cancer but has little to do with breast cancer risk. Some studies indicate that regular exercise (four hours or more per week) or heavy manual labor at work can reduce the chance of getting breast cancer. It is not known why this happens, whether it is due to changes in hormone levels which occur with vigorous exercise, athletes' eating habits or perhaps the different amounts of body fat carried by active and inactive women. This area requires further study, but several hours per week of regular exercise is to be encouraged.

Stress has many different meanings and personal interpretations but usually involves a sense of loss of control or low self-esteem. Making positive changes to reduce your personal level of stress can have substantial health benefits.

Diet

Diet is clearly an important factor in the development of breast cancer and is something which you can change. However, there is no simple remedy to prevent breast cancer in spite of what one reads on the newsstands. A healthy diet would consist of reducing your total amount of calories eaten and reducing the proportion of calories taken as fat to between 20% and 30% of your total calorie intake. This can be achieved by trimming the visible fat from meat, using leaner cuts, avoiding chocolate, avoiding sauces rich in fat or cream, and substituting low fat milk products (skim or 1%) for the higher fat alternatives. Increasing the amount of green and yellow vegetables, which contain vitamin A, and the fiber content of the diet is to be encouraged (see Chapter 36). It is generally felt that drinking less alcohol may be beneficial, but it is not known how much is safe or is too much. A glass of wine a few times per week is probably still reasonable. Ongoing studies are testing whether dietary restrictions later in life can reduce the chance of developing breast cancer.

No specific dietary therapy can guarantee that breast cancer will not develop. Vegetarians also get breast cancer. However, diet is something over which you do have control: make the most of this power, but don't make yourself miserable! It is important to be prudent, enjoy variety and to maintain balance.

Several recent cookbooks provide tasty, interesting, yet simple menus with attention to a new 'lean' life style (see Additional Reading).

Hormones

Moderate use of oral contraceptives and postmenopausal estrogens (over a period of five to ten years) probably has more advantages with respect to general health than disadvantages in terms of breast cancer risk. It is important to remember that the whole person needs to be considered, not just the risk of breast cancer on its own. However, limiting oral contraceptive and postmenopausal estrogen use to less than 10 years where feasible may help reduce the chance of getting breast cancer.

Tamoxifen, an 'anti-estrogen' drug, is used to fight some types of breast cancer (see Chapter 30). Recently, results were reported from a North American study which tested the value of tamoxifen as a method of preventing breast cancer. Over 13,000 women who had five times higher than the normal risk of developing breast cancer volunteered for this study. Tamoxifen was shown to reduce the chance of developing breast cancer and hip fractures, but increased the chance of developing blood clots in the legs and lungs and the chance of getting cancer of the endometrium (uterus). As a result, tamoxifen is not routinely recommended. However, for women at very high risk of developing breast cancer (those at more than five times the average risk), especially if she has had a hysterectomy and therefore does not have to worry about developing uterine cancer, taking tamoxifen for five years may have more benefits than risks. Women should discuss their individual risk of breast cancer and the likelihood of complications from tamoxifen with their doctors.

Raloxifene, another anti-estrogen, has been shown to reduce the risk of osteoporosis. A side benefit seems to be some reduction in the risk of breast cancer, similar to that seen with tamoxifen. Raloxifene causes the same anti-estrogenic side effect of hot flashes as tamoxifen, but should have a lower risk of causing phlebitis and endometrial cancer. A study is being developed to directly compare tamoxifen and raloxifene for the prevention of breast cancer.

Surgical prevention

Rarely, a family may have breast cancer in three or more generations with several members of each generation affected. These families may benefit from special genetic counseling. Much research is now aimed at identifying specific genes that will indicate which women in these families have an extremely high risk of developing breast cancer. The structure of two such genes, called 'BRCA1' and 'BRCA2' were discovered in 1994. Women who have inherited the BRCA1 gene generally have many cases of breast and ovary cancer in their extended families, and have a 70% chance of developing breast cancer and a 45% chance of developing ovary cancer. Women with BRCA2 have a high risk of breast cancer, as do men in the family, but less risk of ovary cancer. This field of medicine and science is changing rapidly.

Surgical prevention (removal of both breasts) is a drastic measure that should be considered only by women with a very high risk (50% or higher) of getting breast cancer and who have participated in counseling and weighed the alternatives carefully. This procedure is called 'prophylactic mastectomy.' If both breasts are to be removed as a preventive measure, then the nipples and all the underlying breast tissue should be removed. However, it is not necessary to take out the lymph nodes. Unfortunately, 100% of the breast glands can never be removed so a small risk of developing breast cancer will still remain.

If a mastectomy is chosen, it may be psychologically advantageous to some women to do an immediate reconstruction. This involves recreating the breast mound (Chapter 35). A popular method is the 'skin-sparing' mastectomy. This involves removing the nipple, areola and all the underlying breast tissue, but leaving most of the skin of the breast. The space created is then filled with an implant or with the woman's own tissue by surgically transplanting fat and muscle tissue from the abdomen or the back. The operation in which tissue is moved from the abdomen to the breast area is called a TRAM flap (from Tissue Rectus Abdominus Muscle) and results in the woman having a 'tummy tuck' at the same time. 'Subcutaneous mastectomy' is a procedure in which the breast tissue is cut out through a small incision under each breast but the nipple and skin of the breast are not removed. Studies have shown that this procedure actually leaves behind nearly 15% of the breast tissue, so the risk of breast cancer is not eliminated. If the decision is taken to use a surgical approach to breast cancer prevention, eliminating as much of the breast tissue as possible is the goal, so total mastectomy with or without reconstruction is preferred.

Routine Methods for Detecting Cancer

CHAPTER SIX

Screening mammography and self-examination can mean early detection

What is screening?

SCREENING IS THE USE OF A TEST or examination to detect a disease at an early stage in someone who appears well, in other words, with no symptoms. With breast cancer, the goal of screening is to detect cancer that is so small that it hasn't had a chance to spread yet. Hopefully, treatment will be less radical at this stage and will give a better chance of a cure. For example, if a woman's cancer is found when it is smaller than 1.0 cm in diameter and has not spread to the lymph nodes, it can be treated with a simple operation that leaves the breast intact and she has a better than 90% chance of being cured.

A small cancer means a better chance of cure

A 'small' breast cancer refers to a lump less than 1 to 1.5 cm in diameter (about the width of your little finger) that has not spread to the lymph nodes in the armpit (Figure 7). Cancers of this size are often too small to feel in a normal breast. If not seen on a breast x-ray (mammogram), it may take two to five years to show up as a lump that a woman or her doctor can feel.

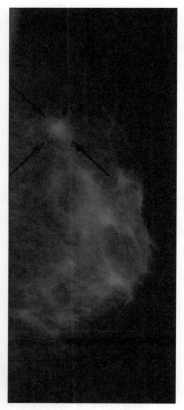

Figure 7: A 6 mm invasive cancer was detected on a screening mammogram (arrows). This cancer might have taken another three to five years before it could be felt. This woman was treated by an operation that saved the breast and her chances of being cured are greater than 95%.

Breast cancers detected and treated effectively at this 'small' size have an excellent chance of being completely cured.

Once a cancer is larger than 2.0 cm there is a higher chance that it has already spread to the lymph nodes or elsewhere in the body. A woman with a 3.0 cm tumor, even if it hasn't spread to her lymph nodes, has a 25% chance of developing a recurrence within five years; a woman with a 3.0 cm tumor that has spread to two lymph nodes at the time of diagnosis has a 50% chance of developing more cancer within five years. Therefore, early detection provides a very real hope for increasing the chance of cure and reducing the number of deaths due to breast cancer.

A 3-step plan for early detection

Effective early detection includes a three-pronged approach that requires the woman's participation. She must take responsibility for learning and performing regular breast self-examination, for having an annual physical examination done by a trained health professional, and having mammography done if she is in the appropriate age category. These three parts are all necessary — no single approach can detect all the cancers and each assesses the breast in a different way.

Breast self-examination: any CHANGE is important

Most breast lumps are not cancerous. Many women develop an occasional non-cancerous (benign) lump in the breast that disappears after the next menstrual cycle. Others have a pattern of lumpiness which is normal. What must be detected are CHANGES in the breasts.

The best way to detect changes is for each woman to get to know her own breasts. You learn what is 'normal' by doing a regular breast self-examination every month. For pre-menopausal women this is best done four to six days after the menstrual period ends. For women who are not menstruating, the breast does not change cyclically, so it doesn't matter what day of the month the breasts are checked. The simplest thing to do is to pick a certain day of the month (for example your birthday) and always do the examination on that day each month.

A breast self-examination (Figure 8) should start by simply looking at your breasts in a mirror to see if there are any changes in the skin or the nipple. Good lighting is important. Put your hands on your hips and press your hips to contract the muscles under the breasts and look again for any changes. Pay special attention to the skin surface. Look for unusual swelling, skin puckering, discoloration or nipple changes. Then, still in front of the mirror, swing both arms above the head and watch the breasts to look for changes.

The next part of the examination is to feel your breasts. This is best done when you are relaxed and lying on your back with one hand raised behind your head. A good time would be in bed or in the bathtub. Remember, the breast occupies a large area on the chest: it extends almost up to the collarbone and has a part that reaches into the armpit. When feeling your breasts, use the right hand to feel the left breast and left hand to feel the right breast.

Feel every portion of the breast tissue by holding the fingers together to form a small sensitive area. Do not pinch the breast between your fingers and thumb. A normal breast always feels lumpy if it is pinched. Using the flat part of your fingers, press just firmly enough to feel the ribs but not so hard that it hurts. Use a circular motion. Check for any differences of texture or

Figure 8: Breast self-examination technique.

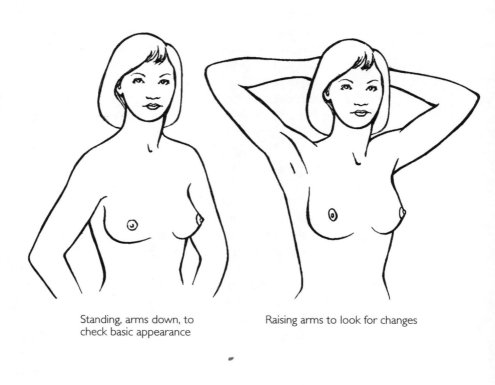

Standing, arms down, to
check basic appearance

Raising arms to look for changes

Using finger pads in circular motion to feel breast

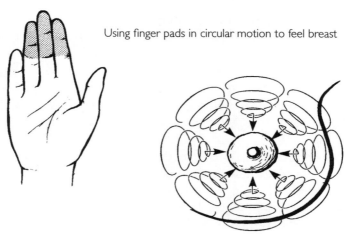

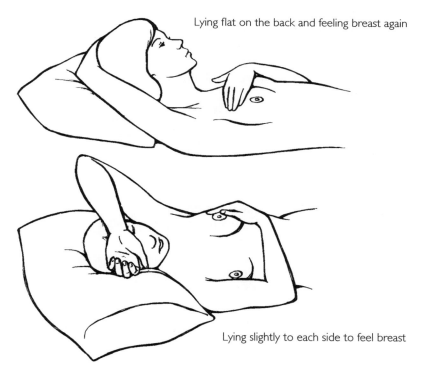

Lying flat on the back and feeling breast again

Lying slightly to each side to feel breast

lumps that are unusual. Divide the breast into four quarters and examine each quarter one by one to be sure that you examine the whole breast. Squeezing the nipples to look for discharge can be part of the examination but it is not essential. Most discharges are not significant and most women have a little clear or whitish discharge.

Once you have felt each breast, concentrate on carefully feeling the armpits where the lymph nodes are located. A new breast lump or an enlarged lymph node should be checked by your doctor.

Breast self-examination is difficult to learn from a pamphlet or by reading a chapter like this. It is best taught on a 'one-to-one' basis. Your family doctor or surgeon should be able to teach you breast self-examination. The Cancer Society, community health nurses and some breast screening centers conduct teaching sessions. You can call the Cancer Society regional office nearest you for further information.

How good is breast self-examination for detecting cancers?

Despite the fact that many breast cancers are discovered by the woman herself, so far, studies have not shown that breast self-examination prevents cancer deaths. This may be partly because most women do not do breast self-examination regularly and do not know how to do it effectively.

Even so, regular breast self-examination is still recommended because some cancers will be found earlier (Figure 9) and treatment may be more effective. Breast self-examination will also give you knowledge about the normal texture of your breasts. New lumps that don't go away should be brought to the attention of your doctor. If you are familiar with your own body you will be confident that a lump is new and can insist that it be taken seriously.

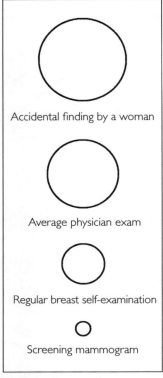

Accidental finding by a woman

Average physician exam

Regular breast self-examination

Screening mammogram

Figure 9: Size at which cancer can be found.

Mammography

What is a mammogram?

A mammogram is a low-dose x-ray of the breast. The dose of radiation is approximately 0.25 centigray (rads) which is about one-fifth the dose of a chest x-ray. It is used very widely for screening large numbers of women who have no symptoms, and it is also used to help diagnose cancer in women who have a suspicious lump (see Chapter 9).

How is a mammogram taken?

The woman stands directly in front of the mammogram machine and the breast is held between two plastic plates (Figure 10). The machine passes x-rays through the breast and

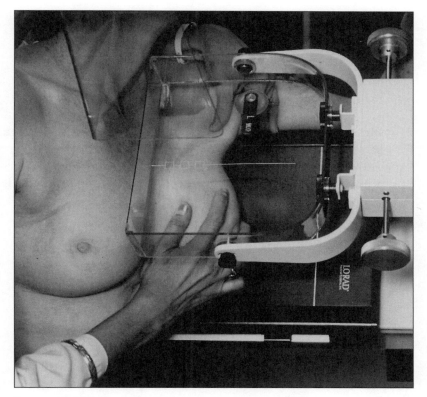

Figure 10: The breast is held between two plates when a mammogram is taken.

onto an x-ray film. Just like the film in a camera, after the picture is taken the mammogram film is then developed. This developed film is 'the mammogram.' The mixed shades of grey, white and black can be interpreted by a radiologist to give information about the inside of the breast (Figure 7).

When the mammogram is taken, the breast is spread out to get a better view of all the tissues in the breast. Unfortunately the pressure on the breast may be uncomfortable but it is brief, about 20 seconds. If this compression causes you severe pain, speak to the technologist taking your mammogram: more gradual compression may help. To reduce the discomfort as much as possible, avoid having the mammogram in the 10 days or week before your period when breast cysts may be more tender.

Does screening with mammography reduce deaths from breast cancer?

Yes for women between 50 and 70 years old

There is strong evidence that mammographic screening for breast cancer can reduce the breast cancer death rate by 25 to 30% for women between 50 and 70 years old. Scientific studies show that the benefits from breast screening are similar regardless of whether women over age 50 have mammograms annually or every 2 years. This means that women in this age group are strongly encouraged to have screening mammograms at least every two years.

No for women aged 39 and younger

Screening healthy women younger than age 40 has not been shown to result in any benefit. One explanation is that the incidence of cancer is low at this age. Another reason may be because breast cancers are more difficult to see on an x-ray when they are buried in the type of breast tissue typically found in younger women. As mentioned in Chapter 1, the breast tissue of a 30-year-old woman consists mostly of milk ducts and glands. However, as women age this tissue is replaced by fat. The breasts of elderly women are made up mostly of fat. Because fat is less dense than ducts and glands, it is easier to identify a tiny developing cancer on the mammogram of an older woman with fatty breasts. Figure 11 compares a typical mammogram of the breast of a 35-year-old woman with that of a 65-year-old woman. Clearly, the tiny new breast cancer (lower) would be more difficult to distinguish from the denser glandular breast tissue in the younger woman (upper).

Yes for healthy women over 70

Although there is not much data regarding the value of screening mammography for women older than 70 years, we recommend its use if a woman has no other serious health problems because breast cancer is quite frequent at this age, and these women may still benefit from the early detection of a breast cancer. Screening mammography may continue to be worthwhile in healthy older women even to the age of 80 years.

'Probably' for women 40 to 49 years old

We believe that women aged between 40 to 49 years may benefit from screening mammography. Studies have shown a modest decrease in the number of breast cancer deaths in this age group: 18% after 12 years of taking annual mammograms. This rate of detection is smaller than that in women over the age of 50. Experts disagree on the value of regular screening before age 50 and on how strongly to encourage screening mammo-

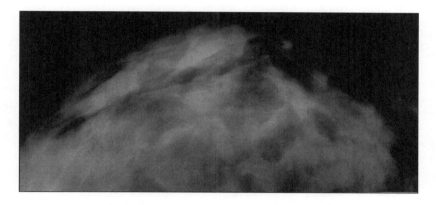

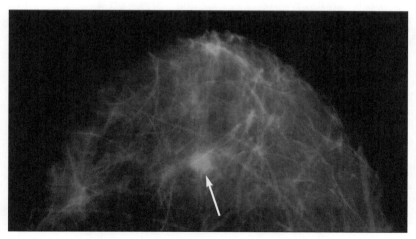

Figure 11: A comparison of mammograms from a 35-year-old woman (upper) and a 65-year-old woman (lower). The small cancer in the central part of the older woman's breast (arrow) would not have been visible in the younger woman's normal breast.

grams for these women. Because the incidence of cancer is lower in this age group it means that many more mammograms will need to be done on healthy women before the curable cancers are found. It has been estimated that about four deaths from breast cancer might be avoided if 10,000 women at the age of 40 had screening mammograms every year for a decade. During that time, many women would be found to have abnormal areas on their mammograms and would need extra tests, including biopsies, to rule out the presence of cancer (Table 4). For other women, cancers might be missed even though they have mammograms.

Each woman needs to consider whether and when to start having regular mammograms. In making this decision, she needs to weigh her personal risk of developing breast cancer and the degree to which she is concerned about breast cancer as compared with the possible need to have additional tests. The higher a woman's risk of developing breast cancer (see Chapters 3 and 4), the more the balance will weigh in favor of starting to have regular mammograms sooner, before the age of 50.

It is important to note that for women aged 40 to 49, there is a shorter time between when a cancer can first be seen on a mammogram and when the cancer shows up as a lump found by a woman or her doctor feeling the breast. This is because the breasts of younger women (and those taking estrogen replacement therapy after menopause) tend to be denser, and the very smallest cancers may not be seen. Therefore, if women aged 40 to 49 decide to have screening mammograms, they should do so annually so that if a cancer is present, it can be detected as early as possible. For women over 50, screening is usually recommended every two years.

Problems related to screening by mammography

The chance of finding an unsuspected cancer on a screening mammogram increases as a woman gets older. For example, among 10,000 women who have a mammogram, between 10 and 120 will be found to have cancer (depending on their age and whether they have had previous mammograms (Table 4)). There are, however, some potential problems with screening,

Table 4   Benefits, risks, and outcomes of screening mammography for women at different ages[1]

| Age | Number of mammograms which appear to be abnormal per 10,000 women in each age group | | Number of women who had a biopsy per 10,000 women in each age group | | Number of women in whom cancer was found per 10,000 women in each age group | | Number of cancers (and %) that were not seen per 10,000 women in each age group[2] |
	At 1st mammogram	On repeat mammograms	After 1st mammogram	After repeat mammograms	After 1st mammogram	After repeat mammograms	
40-49 yrs	1,050	510	123	52	21	12	6 (25%)
50-59 yrs	1,090	460	151	54	48	22	5 (14%)
60-69 yrs	940	370	149	58	69	33	5 (10%)
70-79 yrs	970	370	187	65	111	44	8 (11%)
80+ yrs	960	370	144	76	84	55	8 (11%)

[1] As observed 1993-1997 in the Screening Mammography Program of BC. Source: SMPBC 1996/97 Annual Reports (courtesy of Lisa Kan).
[2] These cancers were diagnosed later by some technique other than mammography within 12 months after a screening visit.

including the need for extra tests and the chance that cancers in the breast may be missed, leading to false reassurance for women. However, the chance of missed cancers and the need for additional tests decreases as women get older (Table 4). Therefore, the balance shifts strongly in favor of doing regular mammograms by the time the average woman is 50. The decision of when to start, whether at age 40, 50 or somewhere in between, should depend on each woman weighing her individual risk, benefits and personal values.

Not all cancers show up on a mammogram

This is a very important point. Up to 10% of breast cancers in older women, and 25% to 30% of cancers in women age 40 to 49 do not show up on a mammogram. There are several reasons for this. Sometimes the breast tissue is so dense that it hides the cancer on the x-ray, other times the cancer may be in such an unusual area of the breast that it is outside of the area that is x-rayed, and sometimes the signs of cancer are so slight that the radiologist misinterprets the film. Of course, the problem with this is that after a 'normal' screening mammogram a woman may be falsely reassured that a lump that she feels is not really a cancer. However, breast lumps should not be ignored just because a mammogram is reported to be 'normal.' A lump still requires serious investigation.

A 'suspicious' mammogram means fear and worry

Table 4 shows that about 6% to 7% of women who have a screening mammogram will be thought to have an abnormality. However, further tests will confirm that the vast majority of these are not due to cancer. These women will undergo further tests, including some having a test called a 'biopsy' where a small piece of the breast is removed and examined under the microscope to determine if it is cancer or not (see Chapter 11). While the few women who actually have cancers are identified, the others endure a lot of anxiety and fear of having breast cancer during the testing process. Furthermore, the women whose biopsies are non-cancerous may be thought of as having had surgery 'unnecessarily' during the process of finding the women who do have cancer.

44

Does mammography itself cause breast cancer?

Since mammography is a type of x-ray there is a certain amount of exposure to radiation, and the fear of causing cancers in healthy women needs to be addressed. The amount of radiation used is very small, and the chance of getting cancer from radiation becomes less as we get older. Therefore, the actual risk of getting breast cancer from a mammogram is extremely small, probably lower than one cancer for every 100,000 to one million women screened. In contrast, between 300 and 4,000 other cancers would be detected in these same women, many at a much more curable size than if screening had not been done. This means that the benefits of having a mammogram every one to two years, especially for women aged 50 to 70 years, are far greater than any risk from radiation exposure.

Other screening methods that have been considered

Although mammography is not 100% accurate, it is still the best test available for detecting 'small' breast cancers. Other tests that have been considered as screening methods include ultrasound, thermography, transillumination, CAT scan and magnetic resonance imaging. Ultrasound, thermography and transillumination have not proven to be as good as mammography in detecting tiny cancers. CAT scan and magnetic resonance imaging, while as accurate as mammography, are much more expensive and time-consuming.

What Do I Do When I Find A Lump?

CHAPTER SEVEN

A *visit to the doctor*

Finding a lump

THE DISCOVERY OF A NEW BREAST LUMP understandably causes tremendous anxiety, but it may help to know that most lumps, nearly 80%, are benign (not cancerous). However, noticing a lump is often the first sign that may lead to a diagnosis of breast cancer. It is important to show any new lump or other breast abnormality to your doctor — and you should expect that it will be looked at in some detail.

What happens when I show the lump to a doctor?

The doctor will ask when you first noticed the lump and whether it has changed, especially in relation to your menstrual cycle. Any previous breast problems and risk factors will be discussed, including biopsies, infections or injuries, and facts regarding your menstrual cycle, use of medications or hormones, and your family history (health of family members).

It is best to examine the breasts of a premenopausal woman a week or two after the menstrual period, but if there is a worrisome lump you should not delay that first visit. During the breast examination you and the doctor are usually alone in the examining room, but you can certainly request the presence of a nurse or bring a family member or friend along for moral support and as a 'second set of ears' to help remember what has been said.

You will be asked to disrobe at least the upper half of your body. Depending on your physician's judgement, you may have a partial or complete physical examination. This may include listening to your chest and examining the lymph node areas in your neck and armpits, both breasts and the abdomen. A pelvic examination is part of a yearly health exam and may be done but it is not essential to the diagnosis of breast cancer.

What happens next?

Depending on what the doctor thinks about the abnormality you may need no further tests. The doctor's recommendation will depend partly on your age. This is a factor that greatly affects the risk of getting breast cancer (Chapter 4). If you are in your teens, the breast lump is almost certainly benign: breast cancer is very rare in this age group. If you are in your twenties, the vast majority of lumps are benign, but an occasional case of breast cancer is seen every year. In the thirties and forties, breast cancer becomes more frequent, and among postmenopausal women there is a substantial possibility that a new breast lump is cancerous.

If some tests are needed, they may be done in the office or you may be sent for a mammogram, ultrasound or other tests. Assessment of your particular breast problem may require consultation with a surgeon, or you may need a biopsy, which involves surgical removal of a small piece of breast tissue for further examination (see Chapter 11).

CHAPTER EIGHT

Breast lumps and other signs of trouble

Breast cysts

MANY WOMEN HAVE PAIN, lumpiness and swelling of the breasts one to two weeks before their menstrual period begins. This is due to hormones in the breast glands that cause fluid-filled lumps called 'cysts' to become swollen and tight. Such cysts are rarely associated with cancer, in other words, they are benign.

Fibrocystic disease

This condition is so common that many doctors feel it should not be called a 'disease' at all, just a 'variation of normal.' Fibrocystic breasts have areas of fibrosis (scarring) and cysts (enlarged milk glands) which cause lumpiness of the breasts that may come and go with the body's normal hormone changes.

As a rule, fibrocystic disease is only associated with a higher chance of developing breast cancer if the cells lining the cysts or ducts show excessive cell growth (hyperplasia) and an abnormal appearance under the microscope (atypia). Chapter 2 gives a more detailed description of atypia and hyperplasia.

Other breast changes not related to cancer

Sclerosing adenosis

Sclerosing adenosis means that there is a lot of scarring and inflammation around the breast glands. This condition may show up as fine calcifications on a mammogram.

Duct ectasia

Duct ectasia refers to widened (or dilated) milk ducts. This is often seen in women who have had surgery for nipple discharge. The dilated ducts can become filled with dead cells and fluids, and may bleed or become infected.

Papillomas

Papillomas are small growths inside the milk ducts. They are benign, but may cause bleeding from the nipple.

Apocrine metaplasia

Apocrine metaplasia means that the milk duct cells have a different appearance when looked at under a microscope. It is not related to cancer in any way, nor is it a reason for concern, but it may be mentioned in a 'pathology report' of a breast biopsy (see Chapter 13).

Fibroadenomas

Fibroadenomas are firm, round, fibrous lumps that are most often found in young women.

Fat necrosis

Fat necrosis refers to a lump of dead fat cells in the breast. This condition may occur after an injury severe enough to cause bruising: after a car accident, physical abuse or sometimes after surgery. A minor bump or a bra that rubs does not cause fat necrosis, so if a tender lump is noticed after a minor injury it needs to be fully checked to be sure that it is not caused by cancer.

Breast infections

Breast infections are unusual except in women who are breastfeeding. In general, infections are treated easily with antibiotics. However, it is important to realize that a woman who is NOT breastfeeding and notices a red, swollen or tender breast may be showing signs of cancer, and a biopsy should be considered.

Signs that may indicate cancer

Breast lumps

Today, with increasing use of screening mammography, many cancers are found before they can be felt. However, women still often find the cancer themselves. Sometimes it happens during the regular breast self-examination, but more often it occurs just by accident. There is no particular 'feel' to a cancerous lump but some women say that they 'knew' it was 'different' from other lumps they had felt in the past. Cancer lumps are usually firm or hard and, although they are usually painless, they may be tender. Sometimes women first notice a lump in the armpit — an enlarged lymph node. Lumps that feel as though they are attached to the skin or also have skin redness are especially likely to be cancerous.

Nipple changes

Crusting, ulceration or eczema (weeping) of the nipple that does not go away in a few days may be the result of breast cancer cells growing into the nipple. This can be due to cancer or to another condition called Paget's disease in which cancer cells grow between the skin cells of the nipple (see Chapter 14). If the nipple becomes inverted (turns inward) it may be a sign of a growing cancer pulling on the ligaments of the breast as it enlarges.

Discharge from the nipple

A small amount of clear or whitish discharge can be squeezed from the nipple of most women and is NOT a cause for concern. Nipple discharge may occur on its own and may be white, yellow or even green. Although this is unusual it is almost always due to a benign condition.

Sometimes the discharge may be bloody. Although this is usually due to a small, benign papilloma in one of the milk ducts, sometimes an early cancer may show up this way.

Nipple discharge, especially with bleeding, should be investigated by your doctor and may require surgical removal of the bleeding milk duct.

Changing breast size and skin changes

Any new change of the breast should be evaluated, especially if it happens only on one side. This may be as simple a change as one breast becoming larger, or dimpling, redness or thickening of the skin or the nipple. These changes are particularly worrisome because they may indicate that cancer has already spread and is blocking the drainage of the breast tissues to the lymph nodes.

CHAPTER NINE

Diagnostic mammograms

What is a mammogram and how is it taken?

THESE ASPECTS ARE EXPLAINED in detail in Chapter 6 and illustrated in Figures 10 (p. 39) and 12 (p. 56).

Several images are often taken

When a new lump is found, a mammogram should be taken of BOTH breasts. This allows evaluation of the lump as well as a routine check of the opposite breast for unsuspected abnormalities. By 'flattening' each breast first horizontally and then vertically within the plastic plates of the mammogram machine, the mammograms will show the breast from different angles and provide more information. Figure 12 shows two views of the same breast. Additional views may be taken to highlight parts of the breast that look suspicious or are not seen completely in the standard views. For example, an image may be taken to focus on the extreme outside part of the breast.

In addition, a 'magnification view' can be used to get a close-up image of an area of concern (Figure 13). These magnification views are taken with special compression plates. Many apparent masses are due to breast glands lying on top of each other — such overlapping glands are pressed apart during compression.

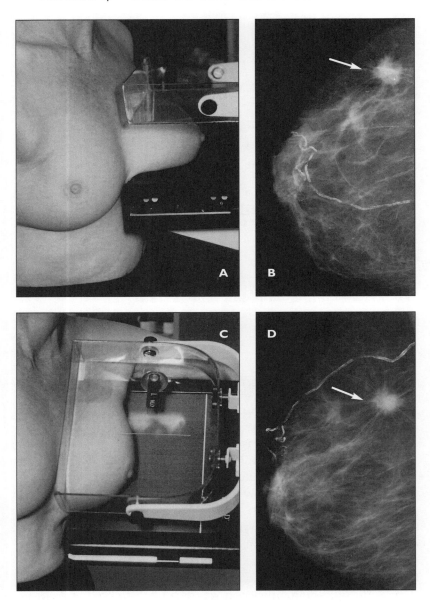

Figure 12: Localizing a breast abnormality requires two views. The first image (B) was made by passing x-rays from top to bottom through the breast (A). The second image (D) was made by passing the x-rays from side to side through the breast (C). The arrow identifies the cancer on the mammograms B and D.

If a mass disappears when it is compressed, it is not a cancer. A mass that keeps its shape is probably real and the possibility that it contains a cancer needs to be assessed further.

Signs of cancer on a mammogram

As mentioned in Chapter 6 on screening mammography, it is important to emphasize that approximately 10% of cancers in older women and 25% to 30% of cancers in women in their 40s do not show up on a mammogram, even when a lump can be felt. There is no single feature on a mammogram that always indicates cancer. However, three features commonly indicate its presence: an irregular dense area not seen in the opposite breast (Figure 13), clusters of irregular, tiny, white areas that indicate calcium deposits, and thickening of the overlying skin, possibly due to cancerous invasion.

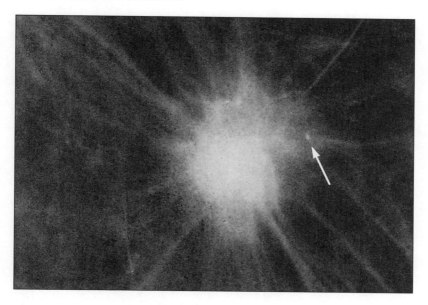

Figure 13: A close-up view shows more detail. The cancer identified in Figure 12 is shown in a 'magnification' view which gives a more detailed 'close-up' view of the abnormality. The thin white streaks extending from the main body of the cancer are 'arms' or tentacles of cancer growing out into the tissues. The small, irregular, very dense white spot (arrow) is a calcium deposit inside a milk duct that is cancerous.

There are many possible reasons, other than cancer, for lumps or calcium deposits on a mammogram. If a lump or calcium deposit is very smooth and round or unchanged for several years, it is not likely to be due to cancer and doesn't need to be removed (Figure 14). However, if an abnormality is new or irregular it should be removed to check if a cancer is present. Therefore, careful interpretation is necessary, and radiologists may seek second opinions from a colleague before recommending a biopsy.

Other information from the mammogram

How big is the lump or cancer?

The mammogram can give information about the size of the lump or cancer. Calcifications, for instance, can sometimes be seen to extend many centimeters from the lump that you actually feel. If the lump turns out to be cancer, this information will be very important in making the decision whether it is feasible

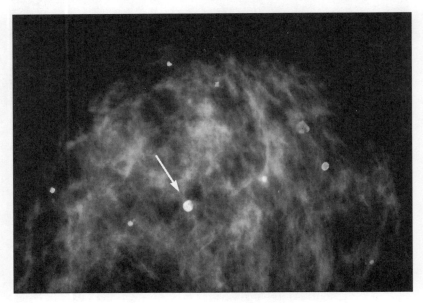

Figure 14: The calcifications (arrow) seen in this mammogram are round and smooth and have been present and unchanged for several years. They are benign and do not need to be removed.

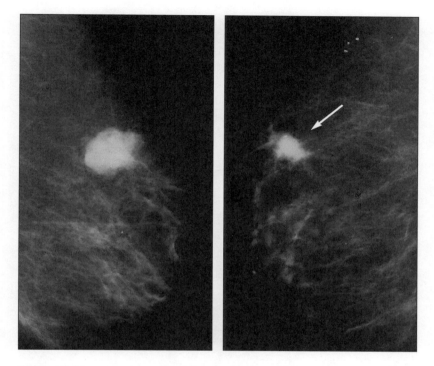

Figure 15: Mammograms of both breasts were used to evaluate the lump felt by a 68-year-old woman in the upper part of her left breast (left). The dense area in the right breast (right; arrow) could not be felt but was also removed and found to be a 1.2 cm diameter invasive cancer.

to save the breast. It is important, therefore, to have a mammogram to obtain this information before a biopsy is done because the breast may feel too bruised or sore to obtain a mammogram after the biopsy.

Is there another 'hidden' cancer?

If one cancer is found it is also important to check the rest of the breast and the breast on the opposite side to make sure that an additional hidden (occult) cancer is not missed. Figure 15 shows the mammograms of a woman who found a single lump in the left breast. A cancer too small to be felt was found on the mammogram of the opposite breast. One or two women in 100 who are diagnosed with cancer will be found to have a cancer in the other breast at the same time.

What are the limitations of mammograms?

As explained above, the main problem with mammograms is that about one out of every 5 to 10 cancers (depending on the woman's age) does not show up. What this means is that if a new lump can be felt but a mammogram is read as 'normal,' unfortunately there is no cause for reassurance. The lump may have been too far to one side to show up on the film, the cancer may have been missed because it looked too similar to the rest of the breast (Figure 16a), or the films, although abnormal, may have been misinterpreted.

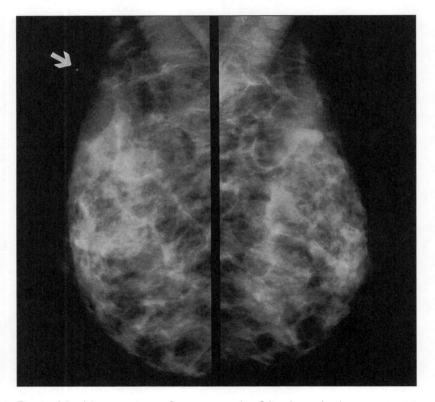

Figure 16a: Mammogram of a woman who felt a lump in the upper part of her right breast. The lump is *not* visible on the mammogram, but the mammography technologist has taped a tiny lead ball on the woman's skin to indicate the site of the lump. It is visible as a white dot (white arrow) on the mammogram.

Another limitation is that although an abnormality may look very much like a cancer or, alternatively, very much like a benign condition, the mammogram alone does not provide enough information to make the diagnosis. If a lump is felt but the mammogram is negative, a breast ultrasound (Figure 16b) is usually done (Chapter 10). If, after the ultrasound examination, a diagnosis has still not been made, a biopsy (an examination of cells from the lump or the abnormal area) is required.

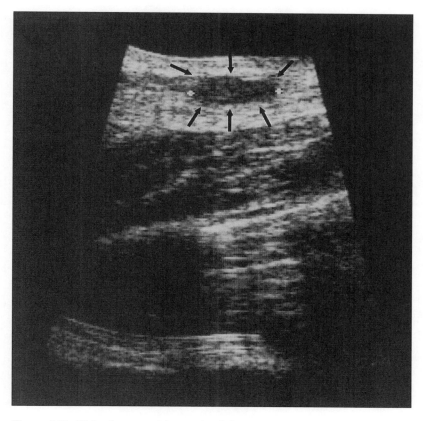

Figure 16b: This ultrasound image is of the same woman as in Figure 16a. Although the lump is *not* visible on the mammogram, the ultrasound shows a discrete solid mass (black arrows) which turned out to be a benign fibro-adenoma. (Figures 16a and b courtesy of Dr. Paula Gordon)

CHAPTER TEN

Diagnostic ultrasound

by Paula Gordon, MD

What is an ultrasound?

AN ULTRASOUND USES SOUND WAVES to assess the breast. This method does not use x-rays. In other words, no ionizing radiation is involved.

The ultrasound machine includes a small hand-held device that is held directly against the skin while the sound waves are transmitted painlessly through the breast. Lubricating jelly is put on the skin to transmit the sound waves better to the skin surface. This jelly is water soluble and washes off easily.

The sound waves are transmitted through the breast tissue and bounce back to the ultrasound machine. The machine then converts the pattern of rebounding sound waves into images which show up on a television monitor as images of the different tissues of the breast.

What does ultrasound show?

The main use of ultrasound is to find out if a lump in the breast is either solid (filled with tissue), or a cyst (filled with fluid). If a lump meets the strict criteria for a simple cyst

(Figure 17), then the accuracy is 100% and additional testing is not required. Simple cysts are not cancerous and do not turn into cancer. They are fluid-filled and easily drained with a fine needle (smaller than the needles used to take a blood test). So, if a lump is a cyst, it can be drained if the woman wishes, either because it is tender or painful or simply for peace of mind, but it is entirely safe to leave the cyst alone.

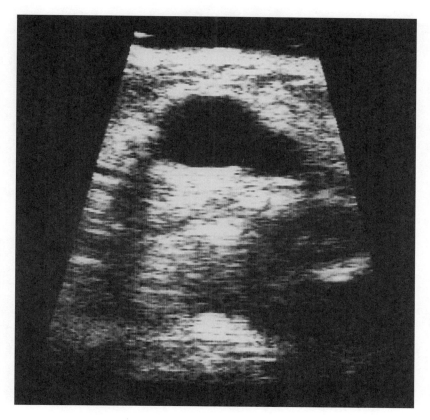

Figure 17: Typical appearance of a cyst as seen on an ultrasound image. The cyst appears completely black and has a smooth, sharp, rounded border.

Not all cysts look completely typical on an ultrasound (Figure 18). Those that are not should either be drained or watched by repeating the ultrasound in six months.

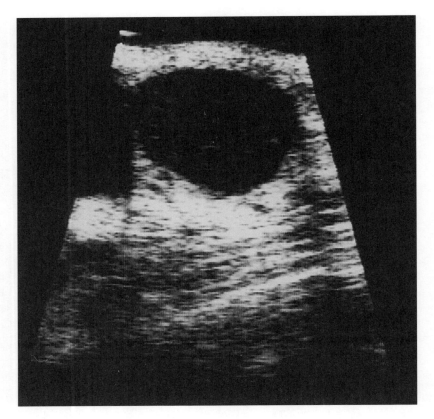

Figure 18: This ultrasound shows an abnormal or complex cyst filled with what appear to be fine white dots. The contents were sucked out using a fine needle. There was no sign of cancer and the cyst disappeared completely.

Most solid lumps are not cancer. Several non-cancerous types of lumps occur frequently, the most common of these being a fibroadenoma (Figure 16b). If a fibroadenoma can be confidently diagnosed by its appearance (and sometimes with a needle biopsy), surgical removal is not required.

Sometimes the radiologist can make a highly accurate prediction that a solid lump is cancer. Cancers are usually solid or partly solid, and have an irregular outline. The clue on the ultrasound that virtually always indicates cancer is when a solid mass looks 'taller than wide' (Figure 19).

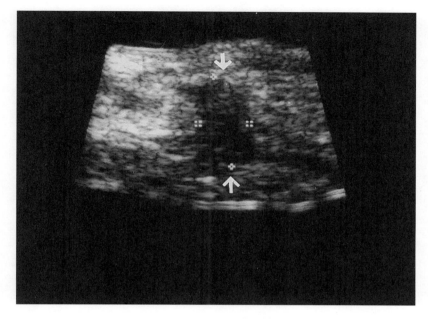

Figure 19: This ultrasound shows the characteristic 'taller-than-wide' orientation of a cancer (between the white arrows). Not all cancers are taller than they are wide, but virtually all masses with this appearance are cancer.

Ultrasound can also be used to direct a needle into a breast lump so that cells can be removed to be examined under the microscope. This is called an ultrasound-guided needle biopsy. When ultrasound guidance is used to position the needle (Figure 20), the placement is more precise than when the needle is placed by finger guidance alone, especially if the lump is deep in the breast. When using ultrasound guidance, a negative or non-diagnostic result is virtually equivalent to a diagnosis of 'not cancer.' However, if there is a persistent, suspicious mass on the mammogram or ultrasound, it should be removed surgically, even if the needle test is benign.

Ultrasound is not useful for screening healthy women in the hope of detecting early cancers: mammography is better at distinguishing the small cancers. Also, the small calcifications which are often the earliest sign of cancer on a mammogram are not visible on an ultrasound.

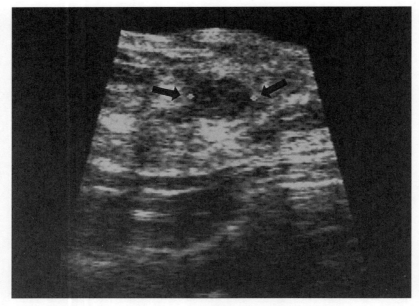

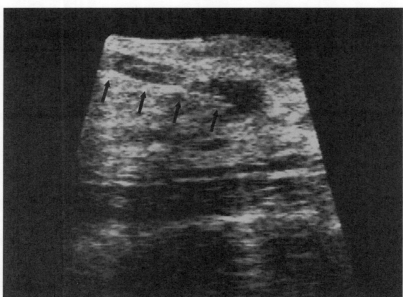

Figure 20: The ultrasound image shows a solid mass (top). The ultrasound was used to direct a needle (bottom, with small arrows) precisely into the mass so that cells could be sampled. The mass was a fibroadenoma.

CHAPTER ELEVEN

Fine needle aspirations and biopsies

What is a biopsy and when is it needed?

IN MANY CASES THE MAMMOGRAMS AND ULTRASOUND (see Chapters 9 and 10) give enough information to diagnose a benign condition in the breast and no further tests are necessary. However, if the diagnosis is still uncertain, then the next step is to take some breast tissue from the area and look at it under a microscope. The process of removing the cells or tissue is called 'taking a biopsy.' There are several ways to do this, some of which are quick and relatively painless, and others which are more complicated and require surgery.

A needle biopsy

A needle biopsy (or fine-needle aspiration biopsy) can be done in the doctor's office. It takes only a few seconds and usually causes no more pain than having a blood test. The skin may or may not be 'frozen' with a local anesthetic. Then, while holding the lump between two fingers, the surgeon or pathologist uses a syringe with a very thin needle to suck some material from the lump (Figure 21).

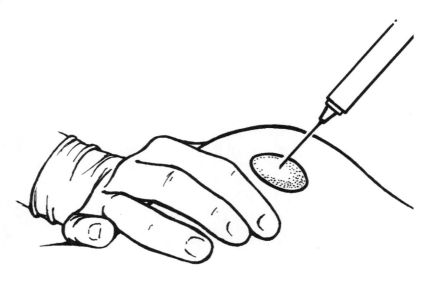

Figure 21: A needle biopsy involves the use of a needle to remove some material from the lump. The needle can be directed into the lump by feel or with ultrasound guidance (see Chapter 10).

If the lump is a cyst

If the lump is a cyst, the fluid in the cyst will be drawn into the syringe and the lump will disappear. No further action may be necessary!

The vast majority of cysts are benign. The cyst fluid may be a wide range of colors: clear, green, white, yellow, etc. Since little information can be obtained from this fluid it is usually thrown away. If the cyst fluid is bloody or if the lump remains even after all the fluid has been drained, there is cause for concern. In these cases, surgery is needed because there may be a cancer that is producing the cyst fluid or the lump. Also, if a cyst appears benign but keeps coming back after several aspirations (removal of fluid by needle), a surgical biopsy may be wise.

If the lump is solid

If the lump is solid, small clumps of cells (invisible to the naked eye) will be sucked into the needle. These cells are smeared onto slides and then prepared for the microscope. The preparation and interpretation of the slides may take from one to seven days.

Based on this microscopic examination of the cells the diagnosis of cancer is quite accurate: if the report comes back as 'positive for cancer' the diagnosis is correct 95% to 97% of the time. However, if the report is 'negative for cancer' or 'non-diagnostic,' it could just mean that the cancer was missed by the needle or that cancer cells, although present, were not sucked out during the aspiration. At least 15% of breast cancers can be missed by the needle biopsy. Therefore, if the lump is solid or looks suspicious, a 'negative' or 'non-diagnostic' report should be ignored and a surgical biopsy should be done.

A core biopsy

For a core biopsy, a needle is used to obtain multiple small cores of tissue about 2 mm in diameter and 1 to 3 cm in length. After a local anesthetic is injected, a small 'nick' is made in the skin and a large needle is pushed into the breast. This method may be more uncomfortable for the patient and requires the use of a special cutting-needle apparatus but provides much more tissue for examination than a needle aspiration biopsy. A core biopsy may be obtained from a palpable mass using ultrasound guidance.

Some centers have a special apparatus attached to a mammogram machine that enables core biopsies of non-palpable lumps to be obtained. The core biopsy needle is advanced to the correct depth under computer-directed control. This technique is called 'stereotactic core needle biopsy' (see Chapter 12).

A surgical (open) biopsy

A surgical biopsy or open biopsy involves making a small cut or incision in the skin of the breast and cutting out a piece of breast tissue (Figure 22). This may take place at the doctor's office or in a hospital, and can be done under a local or a general anesthetic.

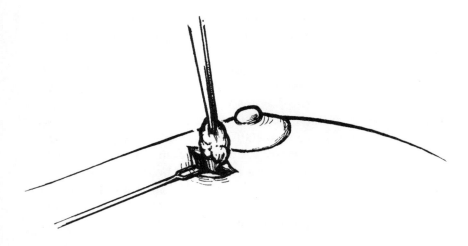

Figure 22: An open biopsy involves making a small cut in the skin and cutting out a piece of breast tissue.

Excisional biopsy: the whole lump is taken out

In addition to removing the entire lump, a small rim of the surrounding normal breast tissue is also removed. This leaves a small scar, but unless the lump was huge it should not form a defect in the shape of the breast. Although such a biopsy can be a frightening experience, it is actually quite a simple surgical procedure.

Incisional biopsy: only a part of the lump is removed

Using anesthetic, the surgeon makes an incision through the skin and removes only a small part of the lump rather than the whole thing. This is done only when a lump is very large and when an excisional biopsy would cause a severe breast deformity or would not remove all of the cancer anyway. For example, when a cancer has invaded the skin or the chest wall, the doctor may do an incisional biopsy to confirm the diagnosis of cancer before discussing treatment options.

Other considerations

Although the biopsy may remove the whole mass, this is just the first step in the treatment plan. The surgeon who will be responsible for the final, curative operation on the breast, if needed, should be the one to do the biopsy. The advantage is that the surgeon can assess the breast carefully and plan the position of the biopsy scar in such a way that it will fit with any additional surgery. The incision should always be placed to give the best cosmetic result and to make as little change in the shape of the breast as possible. The length of the biopsy scar will depend on the size of the lump, but it should not be more than a few centimeters long.

Whichever type of surgical biopsy is done, the specimen is sent directly to the pathologist for a number of studies. If the lump is obviously cancerous, a piece is processed immediately for testing the hormone receptor content (this is related to treatment; see Chapter 30). However, the main part of the biopsy tissue is processed for a detailed examination under the microscope (see Chapter 13).

A frozen section biopsy

In some situations a quick decision must be made about treatment while in the operating room, and a 'frozen section' or 'rush section' is done. This means that a piece of breast tissue is frozen while the patient is still on the operating table and ultra-thin slices of the tissue are examined under the microscope. This takes about 10 to 20 minutes. The problem with this method is that it is neither as good nor as complete as the diagnosis made when the pathologist has more time to examine the entire tissue sample and look at sections from several different areas of the tissue. The diagnosis of cancer inside the milk ducts can be especially difficult to make on a frozen section.

One situation where the frozen section is often done is to confirm a needle biopsy report that is 'positive for cancer' before the surgeon proceeds with the actual operation to remove the cancer (mastectomy or lumpectomy and axillary dissection). As mentioned earlier, the positive needle biopsy is correct 95% to 97% of the time, but this means that in 3% to 5% of cases it is wrong, in other words, the lump is actually benign, and no surgery is needed.

In cases where a diagnosis of cancer has not been made before the operation it is usually best to perform the surgical biopsy and then wait for the pathologist to give a definite diagnosis, even if this takes a few days. Then, decisions about further tests and treatment can be made when the patient is awake and fully able to participate.

Biopsy and curative surgery
Which is best: a 'one step' or 'two step' procedure?

The 'one step procedure' means that the cancer is diagnosed and the curative surgery is done at the same time, usually under one general anesthetic. The surgeon does an excisional biopsy of the tumor and the pathologist does a rush or frozen section to make the diagnosis while the patient is still under anesthetic. If it is cancer, the surgeon continues and does a partial mastectomy and axillary dissection or a modified radical mastectomy, whichever is appropriate (see Chapter 13).

There is no real advantage to having everything done quickly in one procedure, except maybe from a financial standpoint, or for the convenience of the surgeon. There may be disadvantages, as the woman has neither the opportunity to adjust to the diagnosis of cancer, nor does she have any input into the type of surgical procedure that will be used.

The 'two step procedure' is usually preferable. In this case the diagnosis is made first, either from fine-needle aspiration or a surgical (open) biopsy where either the whole lump or part of the lump is removed and a careful diagnosis is made by a pathologist (see Chapter 11). The curative surgery is done as a second step on another day after the pathologist has had time to interpret the specimen. This gives the surgeon and the patient time to discuss treatment options. Since there is no scientific evidence that a short time between diagnosis and surgery is harmful, it gives the patient time to prepare herself physically and emotionally for the next step.

CHAPTER TWELVE

If the screening mammogram is abnormal

by Paula Gordon, MD

What happens if my screening mammogram is abnormal?

IF YOU ARE TOLD THAT your screening mammogram is abnormal do NOT assume that you have cancer! An abnormal result simply means that you need further evaluation to find out if the abnormality is really a cancer or only scarring, cysts or some other problem.

The first step is to go see your doctor and to repeat the physical examination. Sometimes the abnormality can also be felt. Your doctor should compare the new mammogram to other mammograms you may have had previously. A mass that has been present and UNCHANGED for many years does not need to be removed. Often, more mammograms will be taken to provide greater detail of the abnormality (see Chapter 9).

An ultrasound may be used to distinguish between a cyst or a solid mass. Also, a fine-needle aspiration done under ultrasound guidance may provide more information (see Chapter 10).

A new biopsy technique

Recently, a new device has become available in many centers that in future may avoid many of the surgical biopsies that are now done to check abnormalities found by screening mammography. While the breast is held in place between the plates of a mammogram machine, x-rays are taken at different angles that allows the precise position of the abnormal area to be located. Then using computer control, a biopsy 'device' places a core-biopsy needle exactly into the abnormal area. Multiple small cores of tissue 2 mm in diameter and 1 to 3 cm in length are removed (Chapter 11). This technique is called 'stereotactic core-needle biopsy.' It is more uncomfortable than a fine-needle aspiration but provides much more tissue for analysis and diagnosis. The equipment to do stereotactic biopsies is not widely available.

Fine-wire localization biopsy (Figures 23, 24 and 25)

If, after the physical examination, the mammograms and the ultrasound, and in some cases needle or core biopsies, the mass in your breast is still 'questionable' it will have to be removed by surgical (open) biopsy so that it can be examined in more detail. However, if the surgeon cannot feel the abnormal area, it becomes difficult to judge how much of the breast to remove. Instead of going in 'blind,' a technique called 'fine-wire localization directed biopsy' can be used to help the surgeon find the exact location of the lump in the breast.

Before the surgery another mammogram is taken. With the breast still held between the mammographic plates the radiologist locates the abnormality on the mammogram, local anesthetic is applied to the skin, and a hollow needle is inserted into the breast down to the abnormal area. More mammograms are taken to check the position of the needle.

A very fine wire with a tiny hook on the end is threaded down through the hollow needle and the needle is withdrawn, leaving the tiny hook at the end of the wire snagged near the suspicious area. The other end of the fine wire is sticking out of the skin (Figure 24). The patient is then taken to surgery for the open biopsy and the surgeon can follow the wire to find the area that needs to be removed. An x-ray of the biopsy specimen is done to confirm that the suspicious area has been removed Figure 25).

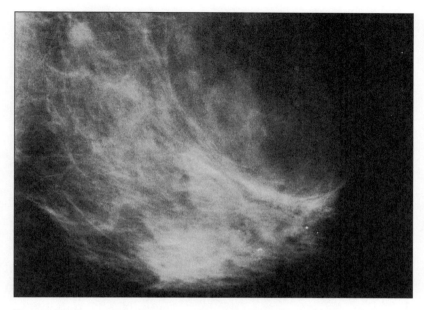

Figure 23: A screening mammogram of a 61-year-old woman showing a suspicious 1-cm diameter dense (upper left) area that could not be felt by the woman or her surgeon.

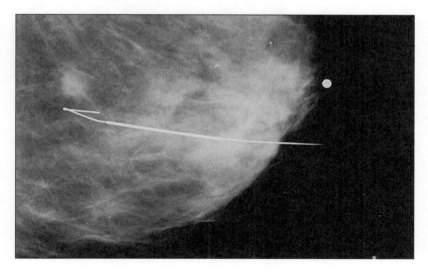

Figure 24: Guided by the mammogram (see text page 74), a fine wire with a hook on the end is placed through a needle into the vicinity of the suspicious area. At this stage the woman goes to the operating room for a biopsy.

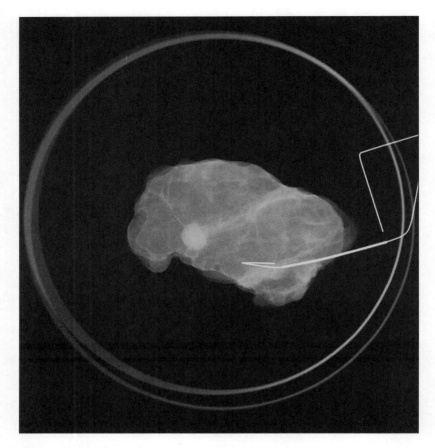

Figure 25: An x-ray of the biopsy specimen removed from the woman in Figure 23. The surgeon cut down along the wire until she reached the tip. She then removed the abnormal area and a margin of surrounding breast tissue. The abnormality turned out to be a 1 cm invasive ductal carcinoma with an excellent chance for cure.

What Type of Cancer Is It?

CHAPTER THIRTEEN

The pathology report: reading the cancer's telltale signs

WHEN A SURGEON REMOVES a suspicious or cancerous lump from the breast, a lot of important information can be gained by looking at the lump itself and examining small bits of it under the microscope (Figures 26 and 27).

In cases where the diagnosis is uncertain, this detailed examination of the breast lump or tissue establishes whether cancer is present or not. In situations where the diagnosis of cancer has already been made, it provides information that helps predict how the cancer will behave in the future. Is it likely to grow back? Where? When? Armed with this information, a treatment strategy can be planned with the goal of blocking the cancer's attempts to grow back and increasing your chance of being cured. The physician who specializes in the study of tissues is referred to as a pathologist, and the pathologist's written summary is called the pathology report.

The three sections of the pathology report

The pathology report contains three main sections: the gross (as seen with the naked eye) description of the tissues, the microscopic description, and the summary (final diagnosis).

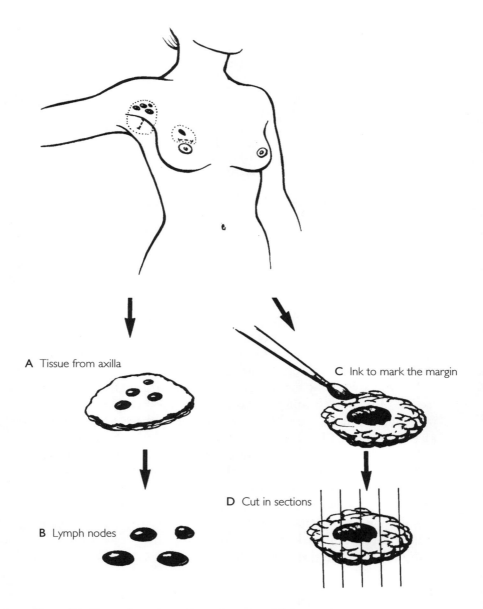

A Tissue from axilla

C Ink to mark the margin

D Cut in sections

B Lymph nodes

Figure 26: Tissue from the axillary dissection (A) is examined and any lymph nodes are removed and counted (B). The external surface of the breast tissue containing the cancer is painted with ink (C) and then the specimen is cut into sections (D).

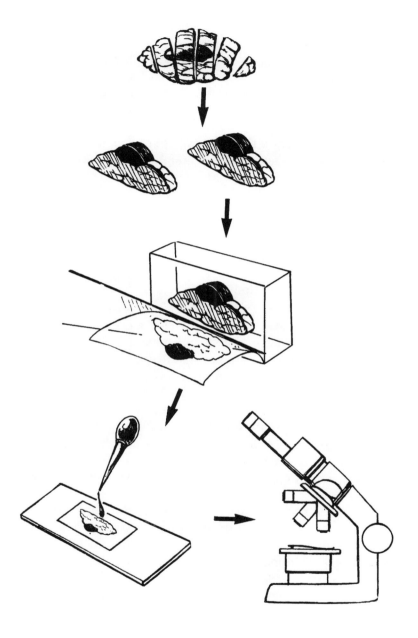

Figure 27: Preparation of a small piece of the breast lump for viewing on a microscope slide.

The gross (as seen with the naked eye) description of the tissues

The pathologist reports on what he or she can see with the naked eye: the size of the lump, and the number and size of any lymph nodes. It is then noted how close the cancer is to the edge of the specimen. This is important: if the cancer is right against the edge rather than being centered within a block of normal-looking tissue, the surgeon has cut too closely to the cancer and there is a high likelihood that some of the cancer was left behind in the breast. If the cancer is large enough, a piece may be immediately frozen and saved for later testing for estrogen and/or progesterone receptor levels or DNA analysis (Chapter 30). Once samples are cut for microscopic examination, the remaining tissue is immersed in a container of formaldehyde and labelled with your name. Specimens are stored like this for years in case further examination is required.

The microscopic description

Under the microscope, breast cancer cells look different from normal cells. The pathologist will write details of the type of cancer, the grade (an assessment of how aggressive the cancer looks), and whether the cancer has invaded the tissues surrounding the main cancer, especially whether cancer cells are seen within the lymph or blood vessels within the breast. Other important features include the presence of dead and dying cells (necrosis), which is a feature of rapidly growing cancers, and the number of mitoses — cells that have been 'caught in the act' of multiplying, which is an indicator of the cancer's growth rate and the amount of estrogen or progesterone receptor content in the cancer cells.

If any lymph nodes have been removed from under the arm the pathologist will report on whether the cancer has spread into the lymph nodes. In fact, the report should document how many nodes were found, and how many, if any, were affected by cancer ('involved' or 'positive nodes'). It should also mention whether the cancer has grown through the lymph node and out into the surrounding fat (called an 'extranodal extension').

Final diagnosis

This is a summary of the results of the gross and microscopic examinations. The process of tissue inspection and preparation of this report usually takes anywhere from two to seven days. The report then becomes a permanent part of the patient's record. The important features which usually influence your doctor's decision about treatment strategy are listed in Table 5.

Table 5 Features of the pathology report that affect treatment strategy

---

The Tumor

Size: measured in centimeters

Type: in situ, invasive, or mixed (see Chapters 14 and 15); ductal, lobular, or other

Invasion: of the lymphatic or vascular spaces

Grade: the degree of aggressiveness

Number of mitoses: the cancer's growth rate

Necrosis: in the invasive component of the cancer (a feature of rapidly growing cancers)

Receptors for estrogen and/or progesterone: see Chapter 30

Extension of tumor: to skin, to muscle, to excision margins

Other prognostic markers: p53, oncogenes, c-erb-B2, growth factors, ploidy

The Lymph Nodes

Total number of lymph nodes recovered

Number of involved nodes

Maximum size of involved nodes

Extranodal extension (growth beyond the lymph nodes): presence or absence

---

CHAPTER FOURTEEN

In situ cancer: Cancer that hasn't invaded or spread

'IN SITU' CANCER IN THE BREAST refers to a cancer that is still within the milk ducts and/or lobules (the milk glands) of the breast. In other words, the cancer cells have not invaded through the walls of the milk ducts; they are in the same place (or *situ*ation) where they first formed.

Ductal carcinoma in situ (DCIS)

The milk ducts become blocked and enlarged as cancer cells accumulate inside them (Figure 28). Calcium tends to collect in the blocked ducts (Figure 29) and is visible on mammograms as tiny white lines and dots (Figure 30). These clusters of fine, irregular calcifications often indicate in situ cancer. If they are present on a mammogram, a biopsy should be done. In situ cancer of the ducts accounts for 20% to 30% of the cancers found by screening mammography. This type of cancer is also referred to as 'intraductal cancer.' Ductal carcinoma in situ, if left untreated, may progress to form an invasive cancer with the potential for spreading throughout the body (Figure 28). In some cases progression can take just a few months, but it usually takes as long as 5 to 10 years.

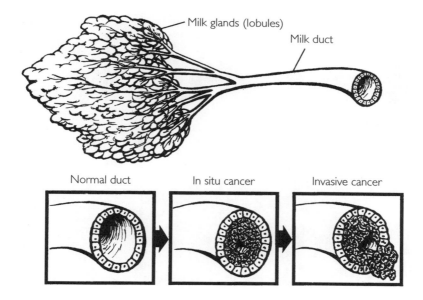

Figure 28: Cross-sectional view of milk duct. The duct may become filled with in situ cancer cells and eventually form an invasive cancer.

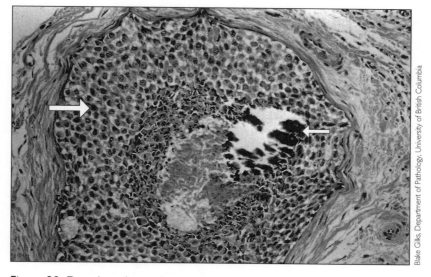

Figure 29: Ductal carcinoma in situ cells (large arrow) seen under the microscope. The dark material (small arrow) is a calcium deposit which has formed in an area of dead and dying cancer cells (necrosis).

85

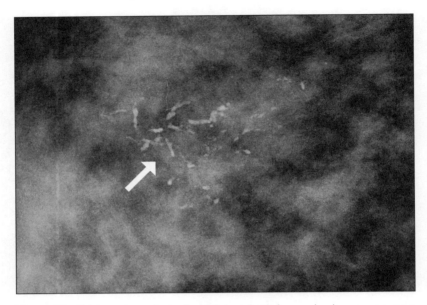

Figure 30: Calcium deposits typical of ductal carcinoma in situ as seen on a mammogram.

Ductal carcinoma in situ occurs as two different cell types, with one tending to progress to invasion more quickly than the other. The first type, which progresses more slowly, consists of smaller, more normal-looking cells. These may be called 'solid,' 'papillary' or 'cribiform.' The second type, called 'comedo-carcinoma,' often progresses to invasion early in its growth and consists of large, irregular-shaped cells which, because they are growing quickly, tend to outgrow their supply of sugar and oxygen. As a result, cells in the middle of the ducts start to die (called necrosis) and eventually the body deposits calcium in the dead cells (Figure 29). It is especially important that comedo-carcinomas are treated effectively. Chapter 20 describes the treatment of in situ cancers.

Lobular carcinoma in situ (LCIS)

Lobular carcinoma in situ refers to cancer cells that have formed in the milk glands (as opposed to the milk ducts) and are still confined there. This type of in situ cancer is often found in women around the age of menopause. Lobular carcinoma in situ is different from ductal carcinoma in situ in that there is a high risk that the entire tissue of both breasts may develop cancer. Therefore, treatment of lobular carcinoma in situ (Chapter 20) must be aimed at both breasts rather than just the affected one, as is the case with ductal carcinoma in situ.

Paget's disease

Paget's disease is a rare form of in situ cancer that can occur in a 'pure' form but it is often accompanied by an invasive cancer. Paget's disease appears as a reddish, itching, scaling or 'eczema' of the nipple caused by cancer cells in the skin of the nipple and areola. Although the traditional treatment is mastectomy, it may be possible to save the breast if there is no underlying invasive cancer. However, the breast must be large enough to tolerate the removal of skin, and the woman needs to accept that there will be a change in sensation and appearance due to the removal of the nipple and areola.

As well as removing the nipple and some surrounding skin, a sample of the breast tissue beneath should also be taken to make sure there is no accompanying invasive cancer. It is not yet clear whether radiation therapy should always follow surgical excision, but in most reports radiation treatment has been added when using a breast-conserving approach for Paget's disease.

CHAPTER FIFTEEN

The different types of invasive breast cancer

What is an invasive breast cancer?

CANCER BECOMES 'INVASIVE' when the cancer cells grow through the walls of the milk ducts and glands into the normal fatty tissue of the breast (Figure 28, p. 85). These cells can also be carried elsewhere in the body through the blood stream or lymph system. It is this ability to invade and spread through the body that makes us fear cancer.

Invasive cancers do not grow like an expanding balloon. Rather, finger-like projections of cells grow out into the normal breast tissue from the main cancer. The body often recognizes these cells as foreign and attempts to mount a defense, which causes inflammation and scar tissue to form around the growing cancer. This is what forms the hard lump which is often the first thing a woman notices.

The finger-like projections and scarring can be seen under the microscope and sometimes even on a mammogram. Figure 13 (p. 57) is a picture of a mammogram showing the typical appearance of an invasive cancer.

Microscopic evaluation of the cancer provides information about its likely future behavior (see Box, p. 90) and makes it possible to counsel a woman about her risks, and about the type of treatment that would best improve her chances of cure.

Table 6 **Classification and occurrence of invasive breast cancer***

From ducts and glands	From other parts of the breast
Adenocarcinomas	Cystosarcoma phyllodes (1%)
Ductal carcinoma	Sarcomas (various types)
not otherwise specified (75%)	(less than 1%)
tubular (1%)	Lymphomas (various types)
mucinous (1%)	(less than 1%)
colloid (1%)	
medullary (1%)	
inflammatory (3% to 5%)	
Lobular carcinoma (15%)	
Squamous carcinomas (less than 1%)	
Mixed carcinomas (adenosquamous and metaplastic) (less than 1%)	

* Percentages refer to the proportion of women with breast cancer who have the specific subtype.

Common types of invasive breast cancer

Ductal carcinoma

By far the most common type of invasive breast cancer arises from the cells lining the milk ducts. It is called 'ductal carcinoma' or 'ductal adenocarcinoma.' When doctors talk about 'breast cancer' they usually mean ductal carcinoma (see Table 6).

In some women the cell type of ductal carcinoma may vary slightly. These subtypes are referred to as tubular, colloid, mucinous, scirrhous and medullary carcinomas. However, their treatment is usually no different than that of other ductal carcinomas.

Inflammatory carcinomas

Inflammatory carcinoma, which also usually begins in the milk ducts, is a particularly aggressive and rapidly spreading type of breast cancer. Fortunately it does not occur often. The cancer spreads in the lymph channels of the breast and skin, causing the breast to become swollen, enlarged and tender. The skin becomes red and warm so that it may look infected. By the time of diagnosis, inflammatory cancer has almost always spread to the lymph nodes.

Trying to predict the future:
How to predict the behavior of an invasive breast cancer

The chance of a breast cancer spreading and forming cancers in other parts of the body (metastases) can be estimated based on certain features of the cancer: its size, lymph node involvement, lymphatic or blood vessel invasion, cancer grade and other factors (see also Chapter 17).

Tumor Size

The larger the cancer, the more likely it has (or will) spread. Breast cancers are classified as 'small' if they are less than two cm in diameter, 'medium' if two to five cm in diameter, and 'large' if bigger than five cm. No matter what size the cancer, if it is invading the skin or growing into the chest wall, muscles or bones it is said to be 'locally advanced' and has a fairly high risk of recurrence and spread.

Number of Cancerous Lymph Nodes

The risk of cancer spreading increases according to the number of axillary (armpit) lymph nodes found to have cancer. If the patient is treated by surgery alone, the chance of the cancer spreading and reappearing within five to ten years is: 30% to 50% if one to three lymph nodes are cancerous; 50% to 75% if four to nine lymph nodes are cancerous; and 75% or higher if ten or more lymph nodes have cancer.

Lymphatic or Blood Vessel Invasion

If cancer cells are found in the lymph channels or blood vessels in the breast the prognosis is similar to the situation of having one to three cancerous lymph nodes.

Grade

Depending on the microscopic appearance of the cells, the cancer is classified as grade 1, 2, or 3. A higher grade cancer (grade 3) tends to grow faster and spread earlier than a lower grade one.

Other Features

Other features are less reliable than the above features, but may be used to provide additional information. These include measuring the number of cells 'caught in the act' of dividing, referred to as the 'mitotic index' or the 'percent S-phase' (synthesis phase). Features such as ploidy, p53, c-erb-B2, growth factors, oncogenes and other new tests may be used in some centers as additional predictors of prognosis.

Any woman who appears to have a breast infection (other than mastitis while breastfeeding) should have the condition checked promptly to exclude the possibility of an inflammatory cancer.

Lobular carcinomas

Lobular carcinomas account for approximately 15% of invasive breast cancers. These cancers are virtually always estrogen receptor-positive (Chapter 30) so are quite likely to respond to treatments that involve altering the hormonal balance of the body.

Rare types of invasive breast cancer

Squamous and metaplastic cancers, which also begin in the milk ducts, have a worse prognosis than the usual ductal carcinomas.

Cancers that begin in areas of the breast other than the ducts and glands are very rare and include three main groups: sarcomas, lymphomas and cystosarcoma phyllodes. Sarcomas are tumors of the 'connective tissue' such as the nerves, fat, fibrous tissue or blood vessels in the breast. Lymphomas are tumors of white blood cells and may rarely start in the breast. A detailed discussion of sarcomas and lymphomas is beyond the scope of this book because they are so rare and their behavior and treatment is entirely different from the other breast cancers.

It is often difficult to tell if a cystosarcoma phyllodes is malignant or benign (they are usually benign). The pathologist estimates the possibility of malignancy based on the proportion of cells that are actively dividing (the number of mitoses). Cystosarcoma phyllodes is usually cured by surgical removal of the tumor, either a wide local excision or a mastectomy, depending on the tumor's size and location. Phyllodes tumors may cause problems by regrowing at the original site or regrowing on the chest wall after mastectomy.

PART TWO | # What are my options now that I have a diagnosis of breast cancer?

An Overview of Treatment

CHAPTER SIXTEEN

An overview of
breast cancer treatment

Is there more than one way to treat breast cancer?

YOU MAY FIND IT CONFUSING to learn that the treatment you've been recommended for breast cancer is quite different from what others have received. An aunt may have had a mastectomy, while a friend was treated with chemotherapy and radiation first followed by mastectomy. Another friend might have had a partial mastectomy and radiation, whereas you may have been advised to have a 'lumpectomy,' radiation and tamoxifen.

Why all these different approaches? What do these different treatments mean? What is the best treatment for you? Part 2 of this book describes the different treatment options and explains why each has certain advantages for different types of breast cancer or for different women.

Figure 31 outlines the usual steps that are followed from the moment cancer is first suspected until arriving at a final treatment plan. This process allows for an individualized approach that will provide the best combination of treatment strategies for your particular situation.

The suspicion of cancer may have arisen from a lump discovered by you or your doctor (Chapter 7), an abnormal screening mammogram (Chapter 12) or some other breast problem.

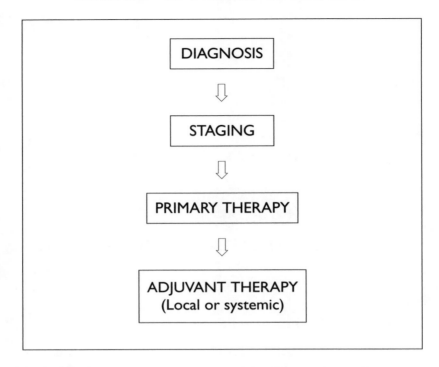

Figure 31: Steps leading to a diagnosis and treatment plan for a woman with breast cancer.

The diagnosis of cancer requires that a piece of breast tissue or a sample of cells be removed and examined by a pathologist (Chapter 13). If a diagnosis of breast cancer is made, tests and examinations will be done to assess the extent (or stage) of disease (Chapter 17).

If the cancer is confined to the breast and lymph nodes in the armpit, as it is in over 90% of cases, then the 'primary therapy,' usually surgery (Chapter 19), is aimed at removing the cancerous tissues. However, new treatments such as 'preoperative chemotherapy' are now being explored (Chapter 27), especially in cases where the tumor is bulky. The important decision about the type of surgery to be used, either mastectomy or an approach that saves the breast, requires your input (Chapter 21).

Once the cancer has been removed, the prognosis of the cancer can be further evaluated by the pathologist's examination of the cancerous tissue (Chapters 13 to 15). A recommendation for additional treatment, called 'adjuvant therapy' (Chapter 23) is based on weighing the likelihood that your cancer will grow back after the surgery against the unnecessary side effects caused by too much treatment.

If the risk of regrowth in the 'local area' (breast or chest wall and lymph nodes) is substantial, then adjuvant radiation therapy is used (Chapter 25). Except for women in the 'lowest risk' category of possible recurrence, additional therapy aimed at the entire body will also be offered (tamoxifen, other hormone therapy or chemotherapy; Chapters 28 and 30). If recurrence in the local area and throughout the rest of the body are both a concern, combined types of adjuvant therapy may be recommended, for example, radiation plus chemotherapy.

The Surgical Options

CHAPTER SEVENTEEN

Staging and prognosis

What is staging?

AFTER THE DIAGNOSIS OF CANCER has been made it is important to determine the extent or 'stage' of the cancer before deciding on the treatment plan. Briefly, a cancer that is small and confined to the breast is at an early stage, whereas one that has spread to other parts of the body is advanced or metastatic. Based on a detailed knowledge of the extent of the disease, your surgeon or oncologist (cancer specialist) can make recommendations about the chances of being cured by surgery alone, the type of surgery that is likely to give you the best possible outcome, and whether additional treatments (radiation, hormone or chemotherapy) will be helpful (see p. 90).

The physical examination

One of the most important investigations is the physical examination done by the surgeon or oncologist. Your lungs, liver, abdomen, back and limbs will be examined for abnormalities. Your breast will be examined and any lumps will be measured. Your armpit and neck will be felt to see if any lymph nodes are enlarged. Not all enlarged lymph nodes are cancerous: the doctor will try to determine this by assessing whether a node feels normal or enlarged, soft or hard, and whether it is movable. If a suspicious lymph node is found, a fine-needle aspiration is done (see Chapter 11). Unfortunately, simple physical examination of the armpit is not foolproof, and sometimes cancerous lymph nodes are not found until surgery.

Blood tests

Blood tests will be done to check whether your bone marrow, liver and kidneys are working normally. Some surgeons also order blood tests to look for 'tumor markers,' which are proteins that leak out of cancer cells and can be measured in the blood. Although these markers are not reliable for diagnosing cancer, they can be useful for checking the response to treatment, especially in cases of metastatic cancer. The tumor markers usually measured in breast cancer are CEA (carcino-embryonic antigen) and CA15.3 (cancer antigen 15.3).

Other tests

A chest x-ray should be taken to check the condition of the lungs and to check for any benign or malignant lung disease. For older women, an electrocardiogram (ECG) may be done to check the heart.

A bone scan is only necessary for women who have a high risk of metastasis to the bones or actual symptoms of such metastases. For example, a bone scan would be done before surgery if the cancer lump is larger than 5 cm or if there are enlarged lymph nodes in the armpit. The same goes for ultrasound examinations of the liver. If liver metastases are highly unlikely then an ultrasound is not done routinely.

Official systems of staging

There are several systems for classifying the extent or stage of breast cancer. The two most common are the Stage I, II, III, IV system (Table 7) and the TNM system (Table 8).

Table 7 **Stage definitions (I to IV) of breast cancer**	
Definition	Average five-year survival
STAGE I	
Tumor 2 cm or less, no metastases, no cancer in lymph nodes	80% to 95%
STAGE II	
Tumor 2-5 cm but not involving skin and chest wall. If lymph nodes are involved they must be movable	50% to 70%
STAGE III	
Advanced local tumor, fixed to the skin or chest wall, or presence of lymph nodes 'attached' to structures in the axilla	30% to 60%
STAGE IV	
Cancer spread beyond the breast and axilla, to lymph nodes above the collarbone, or to distant organs	5% to 20%

One very important point to realize about these staging systems is that they provide just rough estimates of the stage of disease and chances of survival. The numbers are just averages. They do not say anything about the outcome or prognosis of any one particular woman. Each case is unique and other details of your own case, not just the size and location of tumor, are used to help determine your chance of being cured by surgery alone or with additional therapy. In other words, these staging systems, although important, are used simply to provide an approximate idea of the extent of disease to help plan the treatment strategy, but they are far too basic to precisely determine an individual woman's outcome.

The Stage I, II, III, IV system

This simple system defines four stages of breast cancer (see Table 7). Stage I represents early cancer, with a small tumor and

---

Table 8 **The TNM staging system**

TUMOR Stages: (T)

T(0):   no identifiable tumor in the breast
Tis: in situ (noninvasive) cancer only
T(1):   invasive cancer 2 cm or less in diameter
T(2):   invasive cancer 2 cm to 5 cm in diameter
T(3):   invasive cancer larger than 5 cm without skin
        or chest wall involvement
T(4a): tumor of any size fixed to the chest wall
T(4b): tumor of any size invading the skin
T(4c): tumor of any size invading both chest wall and the skin
T(4d): inflammatory cancer

NODE Stages: (N)

N(0):   no evidence of palpable lymph nodes
N(1):   palpable, mobile lymph nodes in the armpit only
N(2):   lymph nodes in the axilla are fixed to each other or to
        adjacent structures such as nerves, muscles, skin or bones
N(3):   involved lymph nodes beside the breast bone

METASTASIS Stages: (M)

M(0):   no evidence of metastases
M(1):   metastases present including spread to lymph nodes
        above the collarbone

---

no spread to the lymph nodes in the armpit. In stages II and III, the tumor is progressively more advanced, while stage IV refers to metastatic disease that has spread to other areas of the body.

Since each stage (I to IV) is rather broad, the survival expectation within each stage is quite variable. For example, for a woman with stage I cancer the average survival at five years after diagnosis is 85%. However, within this category there could be a woman with a mammographically detected cancer of just 0.5 cm in diameter as well as another woman with a 2 cm diameter tumor and cancer invading the lymphatic vessels in the breast. The first woman would have a 95% chance of living free of cancer for over 10 years while the second woman would have a survival expectation closer to that of women with stage II tumors (a 30% to 50% chance of recurrence within five years).

Also, keep in mind that the five-year survival rates in Table 7 are only estimates and your individual chance may be quite different. The 'grade' of the tumor (p. 90) refers to the appearance of the cancer cells under the microscope and should not be confused with the 'stage' of the disease.

The TNM system

The TNM system defines the extent of the cancer based on three features of the tumor: the size/extent of the tumor (T), lymph node involvement (N), and the presence or absence of metastases (M). There are nine possible 'T' categories, four 'N' categories, and two 'M' categories. This system is not as simple as the Stage I, II, III, IV system for everyday use but it is useful for cancer specialists to communicate with each other.

CHAPTER EIGHTEEN

The doctor has suggested surgery: What should I do?

THE OPERATIONS OF TODAY are much less extensive than they used to be. When it comes to surgery, 'more' is not necessarily 'better.' These days there is usually a team of experts who treat the cancer by a combination of surgery, radiation, chemotherapy and hormones. You are also part of the team and have a role to play — learning about the disease, hearing the options, discussing your needs with your family and friends, and coming to a comfortable decision about what you want.

Although long delays are not advised, you should not be rushed or pushed into accepting a treatment plan before you are ready, even if it means requesting a second opinion or waiting a week or so for surgery. You should feel informed and confident.

Do I need surgery?

Having heard of chemotherapy and radiation, many women question the need for surgery, but for most breast cancers, surgery is advisable for a number of good reasons. Some women may be completely cured by surgery alone. For others, surgical removal of the tumor provides better control of the cancer in the breast than radiation therapy alone. In addition, the tissues obtained during surgery provide important information about the type of cancer, size, extent of lymph node involvement and the level of estrogen receptors (see Chapter 30). This information allows the oncologist to determine the stage of the cancer and to tailor any further treatment to your particular case. For instance, if a very tiny cancer is found during surgery, only radiation may be needed to complete the treatment, but if the cancer is more extensive, chemotherapy may also be recommended.

For some cancers, surgery is not the best treatment to start with. This is the case if the tumor is 'locally advanced,' meaning that there is either a very large breast lump or very enlarged lymph nodes, or it is the inflammatory type of cancer. In these situations chemotherapy and radiation may be given first to reduce the size of the tumor. Afterwards, mastectomy may be recommended to remove the primary tumor and reduce the risk of cancer recurrence in the breast.

In the rare instance when there is evidence that the cancer has already spread beyond both the breast and axillary lymph nodes, the initial treatment may include hormones, chemotherapy and radiation, rather than surgery. In this situation, the cancer that has already spread outside the breast is the greater threat, and must be treated first rather than focusing on the breast itself.

Choosing a surgeon

How can you find the best surgeon for you? Usually, one surgeon cannot be singled out who is best for everyone in all circumstances. The ideal surgeon is knowledgeable about breast surgery and current practices as well as being skilful in the operating room. Your surgeon should be someone with whom you feel confident. Don't be uncomfortable about requesting a second opinion if you want one.

Most patients leave the choice of surgeon to their family doctor. This is fine provided you have confidence in both your family doctor and his or her choice. However, you should be aware that family practitioners may not be in a position to refer you to the best surgeon for your case because of standardized referral habits that they use or because they work in a restrictive group practice. Also, remember that your doctor knows the surgeon as a colleague and not as a patient. If you have a good relationship with your doctor or have already discussed your cancer with an oncologist, you may simply need a surgeon who has good surgical technique.

Recommendations by friends tend to be based on the quality of the surgeon's bedside manner. Good information about surgeons can be obtained from women volunteering with the Breast Cancer Visitors program of the Cancer Society or other local support and advocacy groups for breast cancer. The women in support groups will have opinions based on their personal experiences and they will share them with you. You must keep in mind that the best surgeons do not necessarily possess the warmest bedside manner. You should, however, be able to ask the surgeon questions and get satisfactory answers.

Many local cancer clinics have 'breast cancer policy groups.' Surgeons participating in such a group will be aware of current trends and practices and may be more able to respond to your questions.

CHAPTER NINETEEN

Types of breast surgery

Why are there so many choices?

THERE ARE MANY TYPES OF SURGERY available for the treatment of breast cancer. Why isn't there just one operation? Each procedure has its advantages and disadvantages, depending on the situation. The type of operation best for you depends on a combination of factors: the type of cancer, its size and location, your preference, the surgeon's preference, and the policies of the hospital or cancer center where the treatment takes place.

Take time to consider your options

While it is true that you shouldn't delay surgery too long, most cancers have been present for a number of years and there is no need to rush into the operating room by nightfall. A delay of one to two weeks is usually less important than careful consideration of the surgical options. You should understand your choices and feel comfortable with them. There is time for a well thought out choice based on careful examination of the options, discussions with other patients, a second opinion if desired, and an evaluation of your needs with your family and supporters.

Don't assume that you can't understand the various details of the treatment and give up control because of feelings of anxiety or fear. Spend a few days talking with others and thinking about which route is best for you. Taking this time to decide what you want leads to an informed choice that ensures that you remain confident and have some measure of control. In the long run, this is time well spent.

Operations that save the breast

Lumpectomy (tumorectomy)

Strictly speaking, a lumpectomy refers to the operation in which only the lump that is obvious to the naked eye is removed, leaving the rest of the breast tissue alone. However, it is not always possible to see how extensive the lump actually is, so it is difficult to know if removing the lump has removed all of the cancer. Tiny, microscopic 'tentacles' of cancer cells, which cannot be felt by the surgeon, often grow out from the edge of the lump. Since leaving in these tentacles of cancer cells leads to a greater chance of the cancer recurring in the breast, it is recommended that some normal breast tissue around the tumor be removed with the tumor itself, as described in the partial mastectomy (below). A partial mastectomy is often also referred to as a lumpectomy, so it is important to ask physicians to clarify the type of operation they are referring to.

Partial mastectomy: removing a small amount of the breast

A partial mastectomy (also known as 'lumpectomy,' 'segmental mastectomy' or 'wide excision') is an operation that removes some normal breast tissue surrounding the cancer (Figure 32). (In this book we will use the term 'partial mastectomy.') This has become the most commonly performed surgery for the treatment of breast cancer. Studies have found that a partial mastectomy followed by radiation gives a woman the same chance of survival and control of the local cancer as does a modified radical mastectomy (an operation that removes the breast, discussed further on). The fear of the cancer returning should not be the reason for choosing one type of surgery over the other.

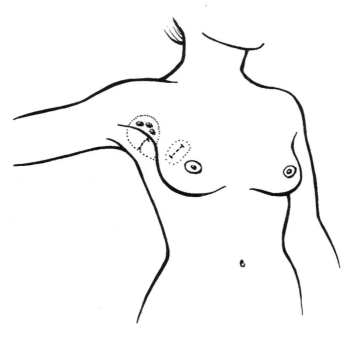

Figure 32: A partial mastectomy involves removing some normal breast tissue surrounding the cancer. The axillary dissection is performed through a separate incision in the armpit.

When the cancer and breast tissue is taken out, careful attention is paid to the edges of the tissue being removed to make certain that they don't contain any cancer. The idea is to remove the cancer lump together with any of its 'tentacles' that extend into the normal breast tissue, but still leave enough tissue that the breast looks 'normal.'

There are several types of partial mastectomies. In the 'wide excision' of a lump, more normal breast tissue is taken than in a lumpectomy. A 'quadrantectomy' involves the removal of a quarter of the breast and skin. The result of a skilfully done partial mastectomy should look very comparable to the appearance of the untreated breast (Figure 33). The area that is cut depends partly on the location of the tumor, the size of the breast, and the surgeon's preference. The goal of the surgery is to remove the cancer but leave the breast as normal-appearing as possible.

Partial mastectomy combined with axillary dissection (removal of lymph nodes in the armpit)

Along with removing the actual tumor from the breast, many surgeons also remove the axillary lymph nodes from the armpit. This is known as an axillary dissection, and may be done at the same time as a partial mastectomy. There are two reasons for doing this. Axillary dissection removes any of the cancer that may have spread to the lymph nodes. Also, by removing the lymph nodes and analyzing them under the microscope, more information is obtained on the stage of the cancer in the nodes, if there is any. This will determine the type of chemotherapy, radiation or hormone therapy that is offered after surgery.

There may be 30 to 50 lymph nodes in the axilla (armpit) but usually, if five to ten nodes are removed this is sufficient to give information about prognosis. It is no longer considered appropriate to do a 'clean-out' since this does not improve survival

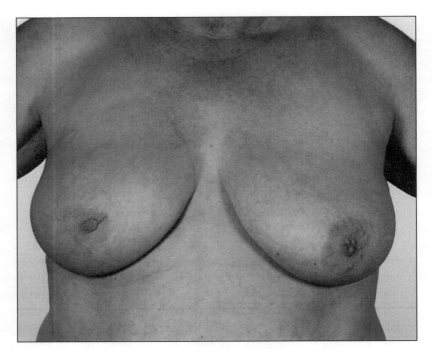

Figure 33: Five years after a partial mastectomy and radiotherapy for a cancer of the right breast.

and does increase the chance of complications such as arm swelling and pain.

An axillary dissection is usually done under general anesthetic and may require a few days in hospital. A separate incision is made in the armpit (Figure 32). Just before closing the wound, the surgeon places a small tube, called a 'drain,' into the area where the lymph nodes were, to collect fluid that would otherwise accumulate. The other end of the tube comes out through the surface of the skin and is sewn to the skin to keep it in place. In a few days, when less fluid is draining through the tube, the drain is removed.

Sentinel node biopsy

A new technique is being developed to try to eliminate the need to remove lymph nodes that do not contain cancer. This technique involves 'labeling' axillary nodes closest to the cancer. A blue dye or a radioactive tracing agent such as technetium is injected into the cancer site in the breast. The dye or radioactive tracer is absorbed into the lymphatic channels in the breast and is then collected and concentrated in the first few lymph nodes 'upstream' from the cancer. A small incision is made over the labeled node(s) and the one or two 'sentinel' nodes are removed and sent for frozen section to see if there is any cancer involvement. If there isn't, then no more nodes need to be taken. If tumor is found, then the normal lymph node dissection is usually done.

Operations that remove the breast

Simple (total) mastectomy

A simple mastectomy is the removal of the entire breast without removing any muscles or axillary lymph nodes. This procedure is useful if the entire breast must be removed and there is no suspicion of cancer in the axillary nodes. For example, for a woman who has a strong family history of breast cancer and who decides to have both breasts removed to eliminate the risk of developing breast cancer (not a decision to be taken lightly), a simple mastectomy is the best operation because it removes all of the breast tissue while preserving everything else, including lymph nodes and muscle. Another situation in which a simple mastectomy could be done is for a widespread ductal carcinoma in situ. A true simple mastectomy will include removal of some skin and the nipple.

Subcutaneous mastectomy

As with the simple mastectomy, this operation has been used to prevent future cancer in a woman at high risk. In a subcutaneous mastectomy, the breast tissue is 'dug out' through a small incision while preserving the breast, skin and nipple. The main disadvantage of this operation is that approximately 15% of the breast tissue is left behind. Therefore it is an unsuitable operation for complete cancer prevention. In addition, results of reconstructive surgery may not be quite as good after a subcutaneous mastectomy.

Modified radical mastectomy

Modified radical mastectomy was the standard surgical procedure for breast cancer for many years. It involves the total removal of the breast along with the axillary lymph nodes, some skin and the nipple (Figure 34). It is called 'modified' because it removes fewer surrounding muscles and lymph nodes than the original radical mastectomy that is now rarely done (see below). A modified radical mastectomy does not remove the chest wall muscles or nerves. This technique is suitable for most patients with stage I or II breast cancer who are not interested in conserving their breasts.

An incision is made over the breast, and the resulting scar after removal of the breast and lymph nodes is long and straight or diagonal across the chest wall (Figure 34). Ask your surgeon how the scar will look and what measures he or she can take to make it easier for you to consider reconstructive surgery if you decide to have it later. A modified radical mastectomy is usually done under general anesthetic and requires a hospital stay of between two to seven days. As the armpit lymph nodes are removed, a drain tube is left in place to avoid fluid build-up.

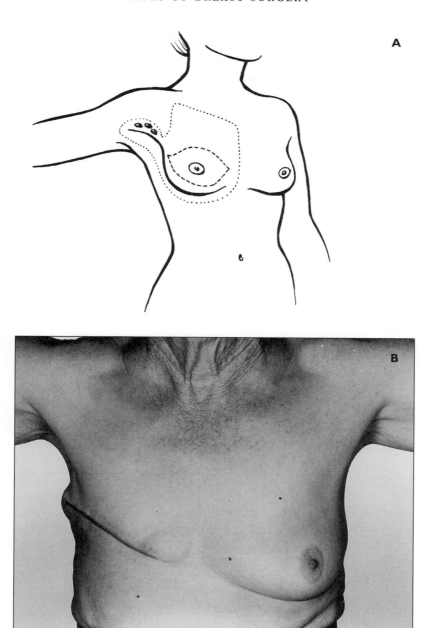

Figure 34: Extent of tissue removed (A) and appearance after a modified radical mastectomy (B).

Radical mastectomy

Radical mastectomy includes removal of the breast, the *pectoralis major* and *minor* chest wall muscles, some nerves, the nipple, the skin, and all of the lymph nodes in the armpit right up to the collarbone. The incision goes all the way from the armpit down to the top of the abdomen. The chest wall ends up looking deformed due to the loss of muscle. Because so much tissue is removed a skin graft is usually needed.

Although these days a radical mastectomy should rarely be necessary, there are cases in which a toned-down version of it might occasionally be considered. An example is a large tumor that has invaded the chest wall muscles so that the only way to remove it completely is by removing a portion of the chest muscle as well as the breast and skin.

CHAPTER TWENTY

Treatment of in situ breast cancer

Treatment of ductal carcinoma in situ

DUCTAL CARCINOMA IN SITU refers to breast cancer that is still entirely within the milk ducts of the breast and has not invaded nearby tissues. Therefore, it has not had any chance to spread to other parts of the body. Chapter 14 provides a description of this type of cancer.

Breast conservation is an option

In the past, the traditional treatment for ductal carcinoma in situ was a simple (total) mastectomy to prevent the progression to invasive cancer. Although the cure rate after such a mastectomy is close to 99%, many women are interested in a treatment that conserves the breast and still provides an excellent chance for cure. Studies have now shown that partial mastectomy followed by radiation therapy is effective and is a common choice of treatment. The procedure for partial mastectomy is discussed in Chapter 19. To remove the entire ductal carcinoma in situ and conserve the breast it is critical that the surgeon plan the operation with a clear idea of the mammogram appearance of the cancer. As well, the pathologist must inspect many samples of the removed tissue to ensure that no invasive cancer is present, and to give an estimate of the completeness of the excision.

In most cases, if the in situ cancer appears to have been completely removed and radiation therapy is given, it is possible to save the breast. A woman who chooses the breast conservation approach requires lifelong follow-up so that if recurrence develops she can receive treatment at a stage when a cure is still possible. About half of these recurrences will be invasive cancers and the rest will be more ductal carcinoma in situ. Usually, if the recurrence occurs after excision and radiation therapy for the initial cancer, then a mastectomy is necessary.

If the ductal carcinoma in situ is extensive

If the in situ cancer is widespread (more than 5 cm across or involving more than 1/4 of the breast), the amount of tissue that must be removed often leads to unacceptable disfigurement of the breast. Also, even after radiation therapy there may be a high (30% to 40%) chance of recurrence in the breast. Since about half of these recurrences will be invasive, with the possibility of distant spread when the in situ cancer is very extensive, simple mastectomy and reconstruction is often recommended to maximize the chances of a long-term cure.

Wide excision (partial mastectomy) alone for very small ductal carcinomas in situ

For some women with very small areas of ductal carcinoma in situ it may be possible to save the breast and avoid radiation therapy. For this procedure to be successful, the cancer should measure less than 1.5 cm in diameter on both the mammogram and in the pathology specimen, AND the area must be removed along with a wide margin of normal tissue AND the cancer must not be the high-grade subtype (very abnormal-looking cells with necrosis) of ductal carcinoma in situ.

High grade ductal carcinoma in situ

Ductal carcinoma in situ that has very abnormal-appearing cells (grade 3; see Chapter 15) and a lot of necrosis in the milk ducts tends to develop recurrences more often than the other types of in situ cancer and also tends to form invasive cancers earlier. These types of lesions are sometimes called 'comedocarcinoma.' To achieve the best control, some authorities recommend adding radiation after wide excision for any size of comedocarcinoma, even if it is very small.

The box below summarizes current recommendations for the management of ductal carcinoma in situ.

Options for the treatment of ductal carcinoma in situ

Wide excision (partial mastectomy) alone is appropriate if:

- The cancer is less than 1.5 cm AND
- Not a high grade subtype AND
- A good margin (≥1 cm) of normal breast tissue was seen between the cancer and the margins marked by the pathologist

Wide excision (partial mastectomy) plus radiation therapy is appropriate if:

- The cancer is 1.5 to 5 cm in diameter OR
- Was the grade 3 subtype OR
- The marked margin was close to cancerous tissue (within 1 cm) as seen by the pathologist

Simple (total) mastectomy is appropriate if:

- The cancer is extensive (more than 5 cm in diameter of calcifications on mammogram) OR
- The margins still show cancer after two attempts at wide excision OR
- The patient chooses this option for any size or type of in situ cancer

---

Tamoxifen is still being studied

Current research is evaluating the use of the anti-estrogen drug tamoxifen in the treatment of ductal carcinoma in situ to determine whether it may reduce the chances of recurrence or invasion. However, as of 1998 there is no proven role for tamoxifen alone in the management of pure in situ cancer.

Treatment of lobular carcinoma in situ

Women with lobular carcinoma in situ (also called lobular neoplasia) have a higher than average risk of developing an invasive breast cancer some time in the future. Overall, the chance of developing breast cancer is about 30% over the next 20 years. The risk of developing invasive breast cancer is related to the extent of lobular carcinoma in situ in the breast biopsy. If there are just focal ('local') deposits the risk is not much higher than for an 'average' woman of the same age. If the lobular car-cinoma in situ is very extensive, the risk of subsequent cancer may be from 4 to 10 times higher than for an 'average' woman. The invasive cancers are about as likely to develop in either breast, so any therapy has to be directed at both breasts.

One course of action is to undertake careful, regular screen-ing and follow-up. Another, drastic choice that has been used is preventive removal of both breasts (bilateral 'prophylactic' mas-tectomy; see Chapter 19 on 'simple mastectomy'). This is done very occasionally if a woman's fear of developing breast cancer outweighs her desire to save her breasts. This surgery may be recommended if there is a family history of breast cancer in addition to lobular carcinoma in situ.

Lobular cancers are almost always estrogen receptor-positive (see Chapter 30), which suggests that the anti-estrogen drug tamoxifen might be able to 'block' the stimulating effect of natural estrogens and help prevent the development of invasive cancers. A large study was recently completed that tested the effectiveness of tamoxifen in women with a high risk of developing breast cancer. The study group also included some women with lobular carcinoma in situ, and the study showed that tamoxifen can reduce the chance of developing an invasive breast cancer. Although tamoxifen is usually well tolerated, it does have some potentially serious side effects such as blood clots in the legs and lungs and a higher risk of developing cancer of the endometrium (uterus). In addition, tamoxifen can affect one's quality of life by causing hot flashes, vaginal dryness, depression or weight gain.

Because of the potential serious side effects, it is not clear-cut whether women with lobular carcinoma in situ should take tamoxifen to prevent the development of breast cancer. Each woman needs to consider her individual likelihood of developing invasive cancer (for example, her age, family history, extensiveness of the lobular carcinoma in situ), her general health (tamoxifen cannot be taken if she has had phlebitis or blood clots in the past), and her other options. Women with a family history of breast cancer and extensive lobular carcinoma in situ and no history of phlebitis may benefit sufficiently from tamoxifen to warrant taking it for five years.

CHAPTER TWENTY-ONE

What type of surgery is best for me?

Does one type of surgery offer a better chance of cure?

THE AIM OF SURGERY is to give you the best chance of being cured of the cancer. Usually, the choice is between a partial mastectomy or a modified radical mastectomy (explained in Chapter 19). Studies show that partial mastectomy followed by radiation or modified radical mastectomy without radiation provide an equal chance of cure and a high chance (85% to 92%) of controlling the cancer in the breast or chest wall. Therefore, your choice of one operation or the other need NOT be based on the 'relapse rate.'

How do I choose the right surgery?

A partial mastectomy is suitable for about 75% of patients. Usually a woman will feel better about herself if she can keep her breast, but there are a number of other factors you and your surgeon should consider:

a) Your preference
b) The surgical issues, including the size of the breast, size of the tumor, its location and the type of cancer cells

   c) Your age and general health
   d) Your ability to undergo radiation
   e) Your availability for regular follow-up visits after the surgery is done.

Your preference counts

Whenever possible, YOUR PREFERENCE should be the deciding factor. A modified radical mastectomy may seem like the better solution for a woman whose breasts are difficult to examine and is 'never going to trust that breast again.' On the other hand, a partial mastectomy conserves the breast and avoids the discomfort and necessity of wearing an artificial breast (prosthesis). Studies have shown that one year after surgery women have similar levels of distress regardless of whether they have had their breast removed or saved. In other words, the diagnosis of cancer causes anxiety no matter what type of surgery is done. Other studies have shown that women who are GIVEN THE CHOICE of surgical treatment adjust to the diagnosis of breast cancer more easily than women who are told to have a particular type of operation.

Surgical issues

Surgical considerations include the size and location of the tumor compared to the size of the breast. If the tumor is large and the breast small, a partial mastectomy may remove too much breast tissue, leaving a disappointing cosmetic result. In this case a modified radical mastectomy may be preferable, with the option of breast reconstruction either later or at the same time. As a rule, tumors smaller than 3 cm can almost always be removed by a partial mastectomy, tumors larger than 5 cm are removed by modified radical mastectomy, and the size of the breast must be carefully considered for tumors between 3 and 5 cm. If the tumor is very large, it may be advisable to have chemotherapy and radiation before the surgery. If the tumor shrinks dramatically, it may still be possible to conserve the breast.

The location of the tumor can also affect the cosmetic result of a partial mastectomy. If it's in the centre of the breast the nipple may have to be removed, resulting in a less satisfactory appearance as well as loss of nipple sensation. If the partial mastectomy is done well, however, the result may be superior to a modified radical mastectomy and reconstruction, or mastectomy and a prosthesis.

About 1% of women are found to have two or more tumors in one breast. If there are multiple tumors within the breast it may not be possible to remove all the affected areas without doing a modified radical mastectomy. Multiple tumors are usually identified before surgery on the mammograms, but sometimes this situation is only identified in the pathology report after surgery. If a mastectomy is felt to be the best choice, it may be possible to do an immediate breast reconstruction during the same anesthetic.

Your overall health affects your ability to undergo radiation

The state of your general health is an important factor when deciding if a partial mastectomy is the best treatment for you. Since radiation is generally required with a partial mastectomy to reduce the risk of recurrence, this type of operation should not be recommended if you are not suitable for radiation. Radiation treatment may be difficult for someone who is elderly or very weak and has difficulty visiting a clinic every day for three to six weeks. Patients who cannot lie flat on the treatment table, or who cannot lift their arms over their head for the radiation treatment (for example after a stroke) will have difficulty with this part of the treatment. Therefore, they may be advised to have a modified radical mastectomy instead.

You would also be considered unsuitable for radiation treatment if it is felt that you have a high risk of severe side effects (see Chapter 26). Some women who have certain other medical conditions should not receive radiation if they have a choice. These conditions include severe lung disease, including previous tuberculosis, or severe heart disease. Women with systemic lupus erythematosus (SLE), scleroderma or ataxia-telangiectasia may have severe reactions and scarring from the radiation so they may best be treated by a modified radical mastectomy. Women who are pregnant should also avoid radiation if possible because it may harm the fetus.

Women with very large breasts tend to get more radiation side effects because of the large amount of tissue that must be treated. Also, radiation should not be given to a woman who has already received therapeutic doses of radiation to the same breast in the past.

Partial mastectomy means regular follow-up visits

After a partial mastectomy and radiation the breast should be observed regularly and carefully to detect early, potentially curable cancer that may recur. You should get to know the 'normal feel' of your treated breast. After surgery and radiation there are often areas of thickening or lumpiness. This is normal but changes in the lumpiness should be reported to your doctor. The best way to monitor your breasts is by a monthly breast self-examination. You should also have a physical examination every six months by a knowledgeable physician, for example your surgeon, an oncologist or another experienced physician.

**Is a partial mastectomy better than
a modified radical mastectomy?**

It is important to understand that in most cases, a breast-saving operation such as a partial mastectomy followed by radiation is as good as a modified radical mastectomy. This doesn't mean that a partial mastectomy is better, but it does allow you to make a choice. You should consider the risks and benefits of both, and your doctors should give you sufficient information and the respect to allow you to make an informed choice.

The advantage of a breast-saving operation is that there is no amputation. This must be weighed against the need for a series of radiation treatments, and more careful and prolonged follow-up. The advantage of a modified radical mastectomy is that the treatment is over at once, avoiding radiation treatments in most cases. If there is a large cancer or more than one cancer in the affected breast, or if certain conditions make radiation more hazardous, mastectomy may be the better option. However, it does mean that a part of you would be amputated. No one answer is always 'right': each person is different. Therefore, it is appropriate and healthy for you to participate in this important decision.

We also recommend a mammogram six months after the radiation treatment is completed, followed by mammograms of both breasts at least annually. It is important that women who opt for breast-saving therapy realize that they will need ongoing close follow-up. If, for geographic or other reasons, follow-up is not possible, a modified radical mastectomy may be a safer option.

CHAPTER TWENTY-TWO

Hospitalization and recovering from surgery

The recovery room

IN THE RECOVERY ROOM nurses carefully monitor you as you wake up. Often, patients are confused for a short period. Also, you may have a sore throat after a breast operation. This is a temporary discomfort from the breathing tube that was inserted in your mouth and down your throat during the operation. The doctor has provided a list of orders, including pain relief and other medications.

Your surgeon may come to talk to you here, although you may be too groggy to remember much. Only a few preliminary findings will be known right away, as the full pathology report is usually not available for three to five days.

Notifying your significant other

There is usually someone you will want the surgeon to contact when the operation is finished, so that person's name and phone number should be clearly written in your chart. If your significant other is waiting in the hospital, make sure it is clear exactly where they are since the surgeon may want to talk to them while you are in the recovery room to describe what was found.

The ward

The type of operation and your recovery time will determine how long you stay in hospital. Most patients go home two to three days after a partial mastectomy and within five days after a modified radical mastectomy. The sooner patients start moving around after surgery the fewer problems they have, so you will be urged to get out of bed and walk up and down the halls.

Pain

After the surgery there will be some pain that can be controlled with pain killers. Everyone is different, so it is important for you to let the nurse know when you are in pain so you can receive medication according to your needs. Some patients feel nauseated after an anesthetic while others may have shivers when they wake up. As well, many of the pain killers can cause nausea and constipation but this is usually mild and temporary.

Drains

If you have an axillary dissection or a modified radical mastectomy, you may have one or two drains in the area for the first few days to avoid fluid accumulating. The drains are removed before you leave hospital or a few days later, depending on the amount of fluid and how long you stay in hospital. Sometimes after the drain is removed the fluid builds up again and needs to be removed with a syringe. This can be done easily in the surgeon's office during an outpatient visit.

Sutures

Some stitches (sutures) may eventually dissolve on their own while other non-absorbable sutures or staples need to be removed, usually a week to ten days after the surgery. Ask your surgeon what sort of sutures will be used. The redness of your scar will gradually fade over several months.

A *note about visitors*

A stay in hospital tends to bring friends and relatives out of the woodwork. Depending on your personality, this may or may not please you. If it doesn't, the simplest way of avoiding the stress of attending a steady stream of visitors is not to announce to anyone other than your immediate family that you are having surgery. If the visiting is too tiring, speak to your nurse and visitors can be restricted.

It may be that seeing people and discussing the situation will be helpful, especially with people close to you who are supportive. Make sure, however, that the visitors do not need more support than you do, and that you do not let the socializing wear you out.

Going home: ask questions before you leave

You are bound to have questions about what you can do when you get home, so write them down and be prepared to rattle off the list when you see your doctor for the last time in hospital. Make sure you understand what you can and cannot do, what exercises you should do to start moving your arm and when you should start them (Chapter 34), when you should see the surgeon again and when you may see an oncologist. Also, make sure you have a prescription for pain killers because you may need them, especially as you get more active.

Dealing with hospitalization

You may find the hospital's admission routine a source of frustration. You may feel that you are answering the same questions over and over again, but nobody seems to be listening. Hospital procedures require that a patient be admitted by the clerk, the ward nurse, and a number of doctors, including the surgeon and anesthetist. In a teaching hospital the list may also include a student nurse, a medical student, an intern and a resident. Be patient: they are listening, but each of them requires slightly different information. The many questions are useful to ensure that any allergies you suffer are recorded as well as the list of any medication you take regularly, and that everyone knows you individually.

Surgical residents

Many hospitals are affiliated with universities and have a responsibility to train future practitioners. A strong surgical training program employs residents to give quality care before, during and after surgery. In a teaching hospital the surgical residents participate in an operation not only because it is part of their training, but also because most operations require two sets of hands. While patients accept that their busy surgeons require the assistance of the residents on the ward, they become anxious when they learn that the residents may be participating in and, in some cases, performing their operation. Although many senior surgical residents have as much experience and skill as your surgeon and may provide superior results, it is your right to expect close supervision of the residents by the staff surgeon. Therefore, it is more appropriate to ask, 'Who is directing the operation?' rather than, 'Who is doing the operation?' A major operation is a team effort in which residents play an important role.

Possible problems and discomfort later on

Most women do suffer some pain, initially along the incision and under the arm. It may last a few days to a few weeks or longer and can be controlled with pain medications. Later on, some women complain of a tightness or discomfort over the chest area which, although mild, is often bothersome and longer-lasting. This is usually helped by physiotherapy (see Chapter 34). The incision usually heals within a few weeks, but may take somewhat longer in women who have had radiation before surgery.

The risk of infection with breast surgery is usually low, but if there is a foul-smelling drainage, increasingly red and tender skin or any fever, there may be an infection and it should be treated promptly with antibiotics.

With any surgery there is a risk of minor bleeding afterwards, even if the surgeon has been very careful. This can result in a hematoma (blood clot in the tissues) which can be very bruised-looking, swollen and painful. Usually, the hematoma subsides on its own, but it may need to be drained if it is large. Aspirin® and several other anti-arthritis and blood-thinning drugs should be avoided if possible in the week to 10 days prior to surgery. You should tell your surgeon which medications you are taking.

If the lymph nodes are removed from the armpit there will be some disruption of the normal lymph drainage. Any later infection in your hand or arm will increase the risk of complications such as permanent arm swelling. Radiation treatment to the armpit may also worsen these problems. You can take a number of precautionary steps to avoid significant arm edema (swelling) and the related pain and discomfort that can occur (see Chapter 34).

After breast surgery many women complain about numbness in the back of the underarm or on the chest wall. This is usually due to nerves being cut or stretched during the operation, and may improve in the months ahead.

Breast surgery is emotionally difficult for many women. Often, it is difficult for a patient to look at her own body, let alone show her spouse, friends or family the scars. As the incision fades and you use your arm, you can begin to heal. A breast cancer support group and a physiotherapy consultation is often helpful to regain your sense of your body.

Obtaining a breast prosthesis

If you have been treated with a mastectomy you may want to consider a prosthesis or breast reconstruction (see Chapter 35). The prosthesis is a soft, somewhat heavy plastic form that comes in many shapes and sizes to match the many shapes and sizes of women's breasts (Figure 35).

Breast Cancer Visitor volunteers from the Cancer Society will often supply a soft, 'fluffy' breast form of cotton that you can wear temporarily in your own bra. This helps fill out your clothes but does not have the weight or shape of your other breast. A fitted prosthesis will help you feel better and walk straighter. Once the initial pain and swelling of the mastectomy has settled and the wound is healed you are ready for a 'fitting.' This is often four to six weeks after surgery. However, some women wait longer since it is important to be psychologically 'ready' for the prosthesis for a successful fitting.

What to look for

Breast prostheses are not one-size-fits-all and just picking a form off the shelf will not give you the best fit. You need to consider the size, shape and weight of your remaining breast to get a good match. The traditional prosthesis is sold with a specially designed bra with a pocket into which the prosthesis can fit. A recent innovation is a prosthesis which directly adheres to the chest wall. It is attached to the chest by strips of velcro which are glued to the chest and the underside of the prosthesis. Body heat activates the adhesive properties of the glue and the velcro strips remain on the chest wall for a week to 10 days. They come off without the tearing or 'ouch' of the usual adhesive plasters.

Additional garments are available such as bathing suits and nightgowns that are specially designed to hold the prosthesis.

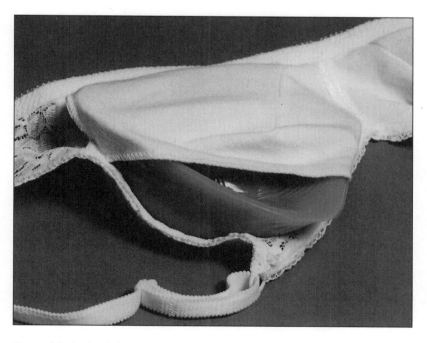

Figure 35: A plastic breast prosthesis in a customized bra.

Where to get your prosthesis

Depending on where you live there may be many or just a few places to buy a prosthesis such as department or drug stores. In larger towns you can find stores that specialize in selling and fitting prostheses and garments to wear with the prothesis. When selecting your retailer, expect the salesperson to offer empathy and sensitivity, but also expect that she has completed training courses in fitting prostheses and that she is aware of the full range of products available today. Your surgeon, support group, local Cancer Society office or nurses at your regional cancer treatment center should be able to direct you to a store. Breast prostheses are a medical appliance so you should check if the cost will be covered by your medical insurance.

Preventing Recurrence of Cancer

CHAPTER TWENTY-THREE

Additional treatment following surgery: Radiation, chemotherapy and hormone treatment

Why is additional treatment needed?

EVEN WHEN THE CANCER appears to have been totally removed, the surgeon can never be sure that he or she 'got it all.' This is because microscopic cells may have been left behind, or they may have spread elsewhere in the body as tiny, undetectable metastases. This is a frustrating problem because only 'time will tell' whether or not the operation was indeed a cure. Until then, the surgery must be considered as 'potentially curative.'

Therefore, treatment is given IN ADDITION to surgery, as a preventive measure, in case cancer is still present. This preventive treatment is called 'adjuvant' therapy. The choices include radiation therapy, chemotherapy, and hormonal agents.

Who should receive adjuvant therapy?

Because we are not able to detect the presence of just a few microscopic cancer cells, each patient's risk of cancer recurrence is assessed based on the surgical findings and the pathology report (see Table 5, Chapter 13).

Based on this assessment, adjuvant therapy may or may not be recommended to a particular patient. For instance, a woman with a very low risk of cancer recurrence and a high probability (more than 90%) of being cured by surgery alone may not be offered any adjuvant therapy. New recommendations are constantly being developed to keep pace with the ever improving understanding of breast cancer.

When should adjuvant therapy start?

Adjuvant therapy is usually started within four to eight weeks after surgery. It is sometimes difficult for women to accept the need for additional treatment so soon after surgery, especially because it requires one to admit the possibility of the cancer returning. Ideally, the concept of adjuvant therapy is best discussed before surgery to give women more time to consider it and come to terms with the reasons for it.

Types of adjuvant therapy

Radiotherapy

Adjuvant radiotherapy is given after partial mastectomy. Although the cancer may seem to have been removed completely, the likelihood of the cancer coming back in the same breast may be relatively high (up to 40% over 10 years without radiation). Radiation to the breast can significantly reduce these recurrences.

Women who have had a modified radical mastectomy may also be treated by adjuvant radiation if the tumor is large (more than 5 cm), if it is invading the skin or the chest wall, or if lymph nodes are cancerous. In this situation, adjuvant radiation decreases the chance of the cancer recurring on the chest wall or in the lymph node areas (see Chapter 25).

Chemotherapy

Adjuvant chemotherapy is given after surgery when there is a risk of residual cancer cells regrowing as metastases throughout the body. Adjuvant chemotherapy decreases the risk of this recurrence and increases the number of women cured. Chemotherapy is the use of drugs given by mouth, or more often, directly into the vein (see Chapters 27 to 29).

Hormone therapy

Like chemotherapy, hormone therapy is also effective against breast cancer cells that may have 'escaped.' The most common form of hormone therapy is a drug called tamoxifen that blocks the effect of the hormone, estrogen, in the body. The connection between estrogen and cancer growth is discussed in Chapter 30. Postmenopausal women appear to benefit from tamoxifen but its use in premenopausal women is still being studied.

Other types of hormonal therapies exist, including reducing the estrogen levels of premenopausal women by surgical removal of the ovaries. Radiation to the ovaries can achieve the same effect and is also sometimes used as adjuvant treatment.

Combined adjuvant therapy

Depending on the type of surgery and the extent of the cancer when it is discovered, more than one type of adjuvant therapy may be offered. Each woman's situation is different. Therefore, one woman may receive both radiotherapy and hormone therapy following her surgery, while another may get chemotherapy alone. When more than one type of adjuvant therapy is used it is called 'combined modality treatment.'

Radiation Therapy

CHAPTER TWENTY-FOUR

Radiation therapy: What is it?

How does radiation work?

RADIATION THERAPY, also called 'radiotherapy,' is the use of high-energy rays to kill cancer cells. Radiation works by damaging the cells so that they eventually die. Radiation will damage any type of cell, either normal or cancerous, that lies in the path of the beam. Therefore, great care must be taken to aim the beam only at the required part of the body and avoid treatment of healthy tissue as much as possible.

Fortunately, normal cells repair themselves from radiation damage more completely than cancer cells do. So, by giving the radiation in a series of small treatments, usually once a day, this lets the normal cells recover between treatments while the cancer cells die.

When is radiation given?

Radiation therapy is used to help prevent recurrence or progression of cancer in one specific part of the body, for example the breast, chest wall or lymph nodes. After a lumpectomy, radiation is directed to the breast to kill any possible 'leftover' cancer cells. It may also be used to treat metastatic cancer in a particular place in the body. For instance, if breast cancer has spread to a woman's hip bone and causes pain, radiation to the hip will kill the cancer cells there and relieve the pain.

The benefits and side effects of radiation therapy are generally restricted to the area being treated. In contrast, chemotherapy agents and hormones are absorbed into the blood stream and affect many parts of the body.

The procedure for getting radiotherapy

The process can be considered in three steps:

a) Deciding whether treatment is advisable
b) A 'planning' visit to the radiation department to mark the area to be treated and to calculate the dose to be used, and
c) The daily visits to receive radiotherapy according to a planned schedule.

The treatment decision

You make the decision to proceed with radiotherapy in consultation with a radiation oncologist (a specialist in radiation therapy). The issues to consider are described in Chapter 25.

The planning session

The purpose of this session is to plan exactly how the x-ray machine is to be directed, given your individual size and body shape, and the location and extent of cancer that requires treatment.

The area to be treated can be marked out by eye or by using a machine called a 'simulator.' The simulator sends low-energy x-rays through the body onto a screen or film so that the target area to be treated can be determined exactly. Very specific information is recorded during the planning session so that the x-ray machine can be accurately re-positioned each time you arrive for a treatment.

Ink marks placed on your body will be used to align the x-ray beam during the daily treatments. It is important not to wash them off until after the treatment is completed. Usually a light dusting of cornstarch will help to keep the skin dry and the marks from rubbing off. A permanent ink dot, the size of a small freckle, is often placed at the center or corner of the treatment area. This 'tattoo' serves as a reference point to avoid mistakenly re-treating an area if radiation is being considered sometime in the future.

Treatment sessions

The amount of radiation you receive and number of daily visits depends on the amount of tissue to be treated, and whether the goal of treatment is to prevent a recurrence or to relieve symptoms. Usually, adjuvant or curative radiation requires anywhere from three and a half to six weeks of daily treatments, whereas when the goal is symptom relief, one to three weeks of treatment is usually sufficient.

What happens during radiation treatment?

Radiation treatments are painless. In fact, when the machine is on, the only thing you'll notice is a slight whirring sound. Treatments may be given from several angles each day to make sure that the entire area targeted gets treated.

You will be in the treatment room for about 10 to 20 minutes. Most of this time is spent carefully adjusting the x-ray machine so that it is positioned correctly. During a typical session the machine is turned on for only one to three minutes per treated area each day.

How much radiation is given during radiotherapy?

The radiation dose delivered to the breast is limited by what normal breast tissue can tolerate. The basic unit of radiation dose is called a 'Gray' (1 Gray = 100 rads). The amount of radiation received during a chest x-ray is approximately 0.005 Gray. For a mammogram it is 0.0015 Gray. In contrast, the typical total dose used to treat the whole breast during cancer therapy ranges from 40 Gray (divided into 15 daily doses given over three weeks) up to 50 Gray (divided into 25 daily doses given over five weeks).

Brachytherapy — another way to give radiation

In this procedure, instead of using a machine that sends out an x-ray beam, a tiny piece of radioactive material is implanted directly into a tumor or into the area where the tumor was removed. Radioactive iridium is the substance most often used, but other materials such as radioactive gold and cesium are also employed.

Under general anesthetic, hollow tubes are placed into the area and stitched into place. This is called the 'implant.' Later, on the hospital ward, the doctor or technician places the radioactive iridium into the tubes, either by hand or by a remote-control device. Depending on the radioactive material used and the dose, the radiation sources may be left in place continuously or may be inserted into the implant tubes once or twice a day for several days. During active treatment the hospital room is considered to be radioactive and visitors are restricted.

Can radiation be repeated at some time in the future?

When giving radiotherapy to a part of the body, the idea is to maximize the killing effect on the cancer while staying within safe limits on normal surrounding tissues. So if a part has been given maximum radiation at some time in the past, treatment of that area must not be repeated. Occasionally, if a fairly low dose of radiation was used and cancer regrowth causes symptoms at the same site, the area can be re-treated. Also, if an entirely new area of the body develops problems from cancer, it too can be considered for treatment.

CHAPTER TWENTY-FIVE

Who benefits
from radiation therapy?

THERE ARE FOUR GENERAL SITUATIONS in which radiotherapy is used for women with breast cancer:

- after breast-saving lumpectomy or partial mastectomy
- after a modified radical mastectomy when there is a high chance of recurrence on the chest wall or in the lymph nodes
- as treatment for locally advanced cancer when surgery is not advisable
- for the relief of symptoms due to cancer recurrence on the chest wall or metastases at other areas such as bones, lymph nodes or the brain.

Radiotherapy following lumpectomy or partial mastectomy

For most women, the best way to remain free of cancer after breast-conserving surgery is to use radiotherapy after the surgery.

Although it may appear that the entire tumor has been removed, thin 'tentacles' of cancer cells have been known to extend more than ten centimeters from the main tumor. For this reason usually the entire breast is treated with radiation.

To avoid unnecessary radiation to the normal structures under-neath such as the lung or heart, the radiation is delivered from side to side across the breast (Figure 36). Women with cancer spread to the axillary lymph nodes may also receive radio-therapy to the lymph node regions above and below the collar-bone (see below).

Radiotherapy after modified radical mastectomy

Modified radical mastectomy (complete removal of the breast) WITHOUT radiotherapy achieves local control of breast cancer for approximately 85% to 90% of patients. However, for some women the risk of cancer regrowth on the chest wall or in the lymph nodes is particularly high, and radiation is recom-mended even after mastectomy. Radiation is recommended if the cancer was very large (larger than 5 cm), had invaded the adja-cent skin or chest wall muscles, or showed extensive spread to the lymph nodes. In these circumstances radiotherapy can sub-stantially reduce the risk of recurrence on the chest wall or in the lymph nodes.

Until recently it was thought that adjuvant radiation did not improve life expectancy. However, several recent reports have shown that radiation added after mastectomy can improve sur-vival. The benefit, however, is modest: a 5% to 8% increase in survival for women with cancer spread to their lymph nodes who live 10 to 15 or more years after the diagnosis of breast cancer. However, the addition of radiation therapy increases the risk of side effects (Chapter 26).

There are differing opinions regarding whether all women with cancer in their lymph nodes should have radiation to the chest wall and lymph node regions. Balancing the potential ben-efits and the risk of increased long-term side effects requires individual consideration of the characteristics and extent of the cancer in the breast and axilla, the woman's current health, the extent of axillary surgery done and whether there are any signs of arm swelling or other complications after the surgery. The more extensive the cancer and the greater the number of cancer-involved lymph nodes, the more worthwhile it is to have radia-tion therapy. On the other hand, if the axillary surgery was

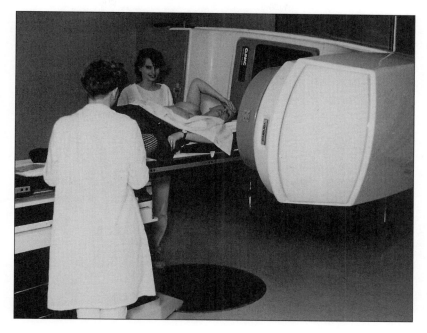

Figure 36: Woman getting ready for treatment in radiotherapy machine.

extensive (more than 10 to 15 lymph nodes removed) and if the woman already has some arm or hand swelling or a history of heart of lung problems, the chance of serious side effects from the radiation may outweigh any benefits. Women with cancer spread to their lymph nodes should expect to discuss these issues with their radiation oncologist.

Radiotherapy for locally extensive cancer

At the time of diagnosis some women already have a cancer that is considered too extensive to treat with surgery, or for some medical reason certain women are considered to be unfit for surgery. These women usually receive chemotherapy or hormone therapy (tamoxifen) depending on their tumor type, age and fitness to withstand treatment. In addition they usually receive radiation to the breast and the nearby lymph nodes. As a result of these treatments, the cancer may shrink to a size that makes surgery possible.

Radiotherapy for recurrence and relief of symptoms from metastases

Radiotherapy can be especially useful to improve the quality of life of patients who have recurrent cancer or who suffer from symptoms caused by cancer that has spread to other areas of the body (metastases). In these situations the radiation works by killing cancer cells, which leads to the cancer lumps shrinking, thereby relieving pain or other symptoms. Pain caused by breast cancer metastases in the bones can be relieved in approximately 75% of cases. When there are metastases in the brain, lymph nodes near the breast or some other sites, improvement of symptoms occurs in about 50% of cases.

Unfortunately, radiotherapy is not helpful when the cancer has spread to the lung tissue or the liver because the dose of radiation necessary to kill the cancer cells in these areas is too high for the organs to tolerate. In these situations hormones, chemotherapy or both are used (see Chapter 40).

CHAPTER TWENTY-SIX

Side effects of
radiation therapy

What radiotherapy does NOT cause

IT IS IMPORTANT TO KNOW that treatments are painless, and, while some people experience nausea, they do not usually vomit, or feel dizzy or lightheaded. You will not lose your hair unless the radiation is specifically directed at your head. Except when brachytherapy is used (a small temporary implant; see Chapter 24), you are NOT radioactive and you are NOT a threat to your friends, family or pets. You should be able to drive yourself back and forth to the clinic for your treatments. Some women even continue full-time employment during radiation treatment.

You may feel tired

Although individuals vary widely in the extent to which they experience side effects, the most common complaint is fatigue. About one woman in three will become noticeably tired. The cause of this is not known, but the best remedy is to have an afternoon nap, maintain a balanced diet, and cut back on stressful activities. After the radiation treatment is finished the fatigue decreases gradually over the next few weeks to months, and it often becomes difficult to tell whether the fatigue is due to the effects of the treatment or the psychological and emotional stress that a new diagnosis of breast cancer brings to every woman.

Emotional effects

Another effect of going to radiation therapy sessions is the daily reminder of the cancer. Many women report feeling weepy, depressed, angry or frustrated. Discuss your feelings with your radiation therapist and oncologist. You will find that it is a normal, common reaction. There may be ways to relieve your sense of frustration by asserting some control over the process by asking questions or helping arrange the timing of your appointments to suit you better.

Side effects in the treated breast

The skin

After a partial mastectomy, the entire breast, skin and chest wall underneath are treated with radiation. During treatment the skin becomes pink, like from a sunburn and sometimes becomes bright red and peels. Afterwards, the skin may appear tanned. Although this tan usually disappears slowly, in about six months to a year, some women are left with slightly darker skin. Occasionally the skin may blister, usually around the nipple or in the crease beneath the breast. Over time the areola on the treated breast may become pale.

It is recommended to keep the skin dry during the course of treatment. A light dusting of cornstarch can relieve itching and help keep the ink marks intact. You may rinse the treated breast in the bath or shower but don't scrub the skin or wash off any treatment-related marks. Pat the breast dry and do not apply any lotions or creams without checking with your radiation oncologist or therapist. If the skin is peeling or blistered, cortisone-containing creams or aloe vera products may be helpful.

Once the radiation treatment is finished, a moisturizing cream will reduce the itching and help to lift off any dead or peeling skin, especially around the nipple, which may remain crusty for several months.

Breast firmness

You may notice that the treated breast will be slightly more firm than the untreated one. Radiation can cause the breast to become enlarged, tender, or heavy with fluid during treatment and for about 6 to 18 months afterwards. This is particularly a problem if the breast is swollen, red, infected or heavily bruised after the surgery. The most comfortable bra is often a cotton 'sport bra' without much elastic material and without lace or seams (Figure 37). While it is important to continue wearing a bra during treatment and for several months afterwards while the breast is still tender, don't wear ones that are constricting or have underwire supports.

'Electric shocks,' burst blood vessels and scarring

It is normal to experience occasional sharp 'electric shock' sensations in the breast or chest wall. This is NOT a sign of

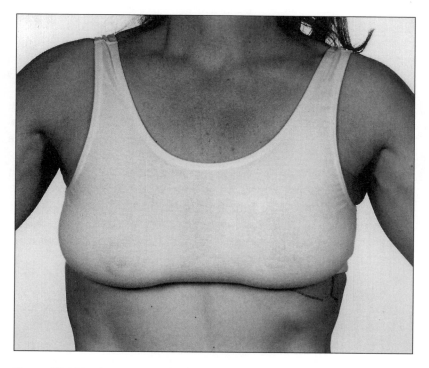

Figure 37: Wearing a supportive but nonconstricting bra is important.

Does radiation therapy itself cause cancer?

Some women are concerned that the radiation therapy itself may cause a cancer in the future. While it is true that low doses of radiation, especially in people younger than age 20, can cause cancer, the high doses used for breast cancer therapy have not been shown to increase the risk of getting cancer later on, at least not for the first 20 to 30 years after radiation therapy. One reason is probably that younger people are more susceptible to the effects of radiation, while older people (those who are much more likely to get breast cancer) are less susceptible. Rarely, unusual cancers called 'sarcomas' have been reported to develop in the treated area. This occurs in fewer than one in every 1,000 women who survive more than 10 years after initially being treated for cancer. However, since sarcomas have also been seen in women after surgery alone without radiotherapy, it is difficult to know whether the sarcomas are due to the radiation or a combination of other factors.

In summary, currently available information indicates that radiation therapy for breast cancer does not lead to a greater risk of cancers later on. Continued surveillance of treated women remains an important area of study.

---

cancer. These fleeting pains are from nerves, damaged during surgery, trying to repair themselves. Red 'burst blood vessels' may appear 18 to 24 months or more after treatment. While potentially unsightly, these are NOT a sign of cancer.

Rarely, radiation may cause severe scarring and fibrosis, with discomfort and deformity of the breast. Women who have a lot of swelling, bruising or infection of the breast after surgery are more prone to develop permanent scarring. Also, a small percentage of women (less than 1%) will develop significant scarring for no known reason.

Side effects of treating lymph nodes with radiation

The throat

If the lymph nodes near the collarbone are treated, part of the throat and the top of the lung will end up in the path of the radiation beam. You may experience a temporary sore or 'scratchy' throat or the feeling of a 'lump' in the throat. These symptoms are NOT cancer, they are just part of the treatment!

The lungs

Sometimes the lung becomes inflamed a few weeks to several months after the radiation treatment is over. This reaction is called 'radiation pneumonitis.' If you develop this condition you will experience a dry, persistent cough, fatigue and, in some cases, fever and chest pain. The pneumonitis usually clears by itself after several months, but treatment with steroids may improve symptoms if they are severe.

The heart

Some, but not all, studies of women who have lived 15 or more years after breast cancer treatment have shown that the women treated with radiation to both the chest wall and lymph nodes after total mastectomy have a small increased chance of having a heart attack. It is thought that the radiation accelerates hardening of the arteries in the heart.

Scarring under the arm

Radiation may increase the amount of scarring caused by surgery in the axilla (armpit). In turn, this will cause more scarring in the lymphatic channels and increase the chance of developing arm swelling. It is important to work at regaining full use of your shoulder, and to pay careful attention to hand and arm care when the axilla is treated with both surgery and radiation therapy.

Scarring on the chest wall

If radiation is given to the chest wall after mastectomy it can cause some firmness and scarring in the skin and underlying tissues. This is usually not very noticeable, but if a prosthesis is used for breast reconstruction (Chapter 35), there is more chance of scarring around the prosthesis. This makes the breast mound hard and it can retract up the chest wall toward the collarbone.

Chemotherapy

CHAPTER TWENTY-SEVEN

Chemotherapy: What is it?

'CHEMOTHERAPY' ACTUALLY MEANS the use of any drug or medication to treat disease. For example, antibiotics are a type of chemotherapy. Today, however, the word 'chemotherapy' has come to refer specifically to the drugs that are used for treating cancer. There are dozens of different chemotherapy (anticancer) drugs. Because they work in different ways, several may be given at once ('combination therapy').

The advantage of chemotherapy is it travels in the blood stream, reaching cancer cells that may be in distant organs. In contrast, surgery or radiation are local treatments that target one area only.

Chemotherapy is used in three ways in treating breast cancer: as adjuvant treatment to prevent recurrence, as the main or primary treatment for advanced (high-risk) cancers, and to relieve symptoms from cancer that has spread (metastatic cancer).

Chemotherapy as adjuvant treatment

The situation in which many patients with breast cancer receive chemotherapy is as follows: they have had surgery and the pathology report (see Chapter 13) indicates that there is a risk of the cancer recurring in other parts of the body. Chemotherapy is added to the surgery to reduce the chance of recurrence from cancer cells that cannot be detected but are presumed to still be in the body. The concept of adjuvant (preventive) therapy is discussed more completely in Chapter 23.

Chemotherapy as initial treatment for advanced (high-risk) cancer

Locally advanced cancers in the breast are considered to be high risk because they are already large when the diagnosis is made. These cancers are usually described in one of three following ways: a) the breast tumor is larger than 5.0 cm in diameter and not easily removed by surgery; b) the tumor is fixed (tethered firmly) to the chest wall muscles, the rib cage or has grown into the skin; or c) there are large, suspicious-feeling lymph nodes in the armpit. Because surgery may be unable to remove the bulk of the tumor or may require the removal of too much tissue, chemotherapy may be given first in order to shrink the tumor.

In this situation there is also a very high risk of metastatic cells outside the breast, so chemotherapy is also important to decrease the risk of recurrence elsewhere in the body.

Usually, a locally advanced cancer is treated with a combination of chemotherapy and radiation. Once the cancer has become smaller, surgery may then be done to decrease the chance of the cancer recurring in the breast. Inflammatory breast cancer (see Chapter 15) is usually treated in the same way.

Chemotherapy for treating metastatic cancer

If the breast cancer has already spread from the breast, chemotherapy may be used to slow its growth, to decrease symptoms that are caused by the cancer, and to improve the patient's quality of life. A detailed discussion of the treatment of metastatic cancer, including the use of chemotherapy, is included in Chapter 40.

How long does chemotherapy take?

Chemotherapy is usually prescribed for a three-month or six-month period. The drugs may be given intravenously (Figure 38) on one day followed by a 21-day drug-free 'rest period' and then repeated. Alternatively, a combination of oral and intravenous drugs may be given for a week or two followed by a two-week rest period. This allows for the maximum cancer-killing effect of the drugs to occur while permitting the body's blood cell counts to return to normal levels during the rest periods (see Chapter 29 on side effects of chemotherapy).

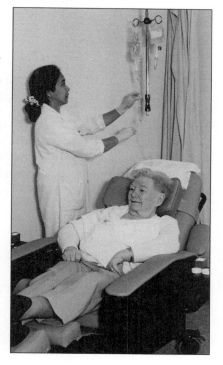

Figure 38: Getting ready for chemotherapy.

"But I've heard 'horror stories' about chemotherapy!"

Chemotherapy has a bad name due to the severe side effects women used to experience when these drugs were first being developed. Because of these problems, a number of new drugs have since been developed that control or eliminate many of these side effects. They are given at the same time as the chemotherapy drugs, improving the patient's well-being while the chemotherapy goes to work on the cancer cells.

Fear also stems from patients not having a clear idea WHY chemotherapy is being given. If chemotherapy is recommended as a part of your treatment, it is important for you to understand clearly the reasons for it or to ask the following questions:

- Why is the oncologist suggesting it?
- What are the goals of the chemotherapy treatment program?
- How long will the treatment take?
- What do I do if I have side effects?
- What are the expected side effects?
- What chemotherapy drugs are being prescribed?

Once you understand the reasons behind the oncologist's choice of chemotherapy, and you know what to expect, it is easier to accept some side effects knowing that the treatment is the best possible choice for your particular situation in aiming for a cure.

CHAPTER TWENTY-EIGHT

Who benefits from chemotherapy?

ADJUVANT CHEMOTHERAPY is treatment given IN ADDITION to surgery and radiation when there is a fairly high risk of the cancer recurring. The reason that chemotherapy isn't simply given to everyone is that there are side effects to the therapy, so this must be balanced against the possibility of receiving benefit from these drugs.

The risk of cancer recurrence varies with many factors, some of which we understand and some which we don't. Table 9 groups patients into broad categories of low, medium, and high risk, which makes it easier to understand the types of therapy offered to different patients.

Recommendations for adjuvant chemotherapy

Adjuvant chemotherapy is recommended if one or more of the following situations is present:

- axillary lymph nodes containing cancer cells
- tumors more than 1 cm in size and high grade (grade 3)
- tumors more than 2 cm in size and low or moderate grade (grades 1 and 2)
- tumors with cancer cells that have invaded the lymphatic or vascular channels of the breast.

Chemotherapy may be recommended more frequently when tumors are estrogen receptor-negative, as they respond less well to hormonal therapy.

For a number of years there were no studies that showed chemotherapy to be beneficial to postmenopausal women or women over the age of 50. Now it appears that chemotherapy can decrease the number of deaths from breast cancer in some groups of women over the age of 50. The benefit of the chemotherapy depends upon the extent of the cancer and the tumor's estrogen receptors. However, it must also be recognized that older women may not tolerate chemotherapy as well. Considering all these factors, women may be offered chemotherapy if their cancer has moderate or high-risk features (see Table 9)

Table 9 **Basis for recommendations for adjuvant chemotherapy**		
Lowest risk (10% risk of recurrence after 10 years)	Moderate risk (25-60% risk of recurrence after 10 years)	Extreme risk (75-90% risk of recurrence after 10 years)
All of:	Any *one* of:	Any *one* of:
Tumor less than 1 cm	Tumor more than 2 cm or more than 1 cm and grade 3	Tumor more than 5 cm with cancerous lymph nodes
plus	and/or	and/or
No cancer in nodes	Nodes contain cancer	More than 10 nodes with cancer
plus	and/or	and/or
No invasion into lymphatic or blood vessels of the breast	Invasion of lymphatic or blood vessels of the breast	Invasion into skin or chest wall
		and/or
		Inflammatory cancer
Treatment recommendations for each group*		
No adjuvant chemotherapy	Adjuvant chemotherapy	Intensive adjuvant chemotherapy
*Varies with age.		

such as a large number of lymph nodes containing cancer, a large tumor (more than 5 cm), locally advanced cancer, or a high-risk cancer that will not respond well to hormone therapy.

Any recommendation for chemotherapy must be made after carefully considering the woman's general health.

Why is chemotherapy recommended for these women?

Cancer-involved lymph nodes

Cancerous lymph nodes in the armpit indicate a moderate or high risk of cancer recurrence. Surgery alone will cure only a minority of these women because the cancer cells have usually escaped outside the breast before surgery.

Unfortunately, chemotherapy is not a guarantee. Approximately three women in ten will have a long-term benefit from chemotherapy when it is included with surgery and radiotherapy. However, these numbers are very general and don't tell the whole story: women with few cancer-involved lymph nodes have fewer recurrences than women who have many nodes involved. Also, newer chemotherapy programs may be more effective than the old ones used in older studies, so today more women may be cured than in the past.

Since there is no reliable way of knowing exactly which women will be cured by chemotherapy, it is recommended for all premenopausal women with cancerous lymph nodes of the armpit and may also benefit postmenopausal women.

What about patients whose lymph nodes are free of cancer?

Approximately seven out of ten women with no cancer in their lymph nodes will be cured by surgery and radiation. However, in the other three, breast cancer will recur even though the lymph nodes appeared to be normal in the pathology specimen.

This is when it becomes important to look at other risk factors that may help identify women at a high risk of relapse who could benefit from adjuvant chemotherapy. The pathology report contains valuable information about the cancer (see Chapter 13) and its possibility of recurrence, and should be used in making the decision of whether or not to recommend chemotherapy.

Cancer invading the lymphatics and veins of the breast

If the pathologist sees cancer cells in the lymphatic channels or veins or nerves of the breast, this also increases the risk of the cancer coming back. Therefore, in some treatment centers, adjuvant chemotherapy is recommended if the pathology report describes cancer cells in these areas.

A large cancer

The size of the cancer is very important. A 1.0 cm cancer is made up of about one billion cells. The larger the cancer, the higher the risk that some of these cancer cells will have escaped from the main tumor and will be growing outside the segment removed by surgery.

Grade of the cancer

Studies have shown that cancers that look aggressive under the microscope (grade 3, see page 90) may recur more frequently. Women with grade 3 cancers that are greater than 1 cm in size may benefit from chemotherapy.

When hormone therapy is less likely to work

In some cases, women with small tumors that are estrogen receptor-negative (poor responders to hormone therapy) may be considered to be at high enough risk of recurrence to consider adjuvant chemotherapy.

What's best for you

As the understanding of breast cancer improves there will be changes in the recommended treatment. As well, treatment policies may vary somewhat in different centers. Apart from these changes, what is important is for you to understand why chemotherapy has or hasn't been chosen for your particular case, and to be confident that the best possible choice of treatment has been made.

CHAPTER TWENTY-NINE

Side effects of chemotherapy

Why are there side effects?

ALL DRUGS, EVEN ANTIBIOTICS or headache tablets, have potential side effects. What counts is that the beneficial effects of a drug outweigh the problems or discomforts of its side effects. Knowing that a particular drug or combination of drugs can effectively destroy the tumor, you may be more willing to tolerate the side effects, especially if they're temporary.

It is important to be aware of possible side effects BEFORE you begin treatment and to discuss them with your doctor. This may make the chemotherapy process less mysterious and frightening, and allow you to decide for yourself whether the benefits warrant the side effects.

Although a number of side effects are predictable, others are not. For example, some chemotherapy drugs always cause hair loss while other drugs rarely affect the hair. Different people can also have different reactions to the same drug. In the last few years a number of drugs have become available which have decreased the most feared side effects — nausea and vomiting.

Drug names and drug combinations

An important point to note about drug names is that all drugs have two names: a 'chemical' or 'generic' name, and a brand name. For example, headache tablets have brand names such as Aspirin® and Tylenol®, but the chemical name for Aspirin® is acetylsalicylic acid and that of Tylenol® is acetaminophen. When you are discussing a particular drug with your doctor, ask him or her to tell you both the chemical name and the brand name (write them down). Since the two names are often referred to interchangeably, being aware of both will avoid confusion.

Different chemotherapy drugs work in different ways. To take maximum advantage of this, the drugs are often given in combinations — attacking on all fronts. Because certain combinations are used frequently, you may see them referred to as abbreviations. Some typical examples are:

- AC — Adriamycin® and cyclophosphamide
- CMF — cyclophosphamide, methotrexate and 5-fluorouracil (5-FU)
- CAF (or FAC) — cyclophosphamide, Adriamycin® and 5-FU
- CEF (or FEC) — cyclophosphamide, epirubicin and 5-FU.

All of the above drug names are chemical (generic) names except for Adriamycin® (its chemical name is doxorubicin).

The side effects

Hair loss

Losing your hair is often the most difficult part of chemotherapy. At the doses used, some of the drugs such as doxorubicin (Adriamycin®) cause baldness for everyone. Other drugs such as cyclophosphamide (Cytoxan®) may cause thinning or total hair loss.

Hair loss occurs because the chemotherapy slows down the rapidly dividing cells of the roots of the hair. Thinning usually begins about two weeks after the first dose of chemotherapy. You will notice that you are shedding in the shower, on your brush, and on your pillow. The hair breaks at or near the skin, so the scalp may be tender. The chemotherapy may also cause thinning of the hair on the rest of your body, including your eye-brows, eyelashes, arms, legs and pubic hair. The hair ALWAYS grows back, sometimes even during the chemotherapy, and it is usually already a few inches long by the third month after finishing the drugs.

Hair loss is the most upsetting event for both women and men: it is a public symbol of your cancer. Unfortunately in most situations it cannot be avoided. Fortunately it is temporary. Buy a wig before it happens and take it to your hairdresser to get it styled so you are prepared. You can also wear hats, turbans and scarves.

Although there have been attempts to decrease hair loss by scalp hypothermia (cold packs on the scalp) or electrical stimulation of the scalp, these are generally uncomfortable and ineffective. Furthermore, as the cold decreases blood flow to the area, many doctors are concerned that by decreasing the blood flow they also decrease the chemotherapy delivered to that area and they may be leaving a potential cancer site untreated.

Infection

White blood cells in the blood stream protect the body from infection. After each injection, many chemotherapy drugs reduce the white blood cell count. If it drops too much your body's defense mechanisms are low and you have a higher risk of getting an infection.

How can you protect yourself? You don't need to become a hermit but you should take precautions: avoid crowds and contagious diseases such as chickenpox, wash hands frequently, practice good skin care with frequent showers or baths, use a soft toothbrush, use an electric shaver rather than a razor, pay careful attention to hemorrhoids, and be on the alert for any signs of an infection. If you get a fever, sweats, chills, a cough with yellow sputum, burning urine, a sore that will not heal, diarrhea or any signs of an infection, you should call your doctor immediately so antibiotics can be prescribed. It is rare that you would need hospitalization, but oral antibiotics may be required for about five to seven days until your white blood cells recover.

The white cell count usually recovers about 21 days after chemotherapy, which is why most courses of chemotherapy are given in sessions separated by three-week 'holidays.' If your white cell count hasn't recovered enough to make it safe to give another dose of chemotherapy according to the schedule, then treatment will be delayed or the doses will be reduced.

A hormone called 'granulocyte colony stimulating factor' (G-CSF, Neupogen®, Filgrastim®) may be prescribed if you have problems with infection or a very low white blood cell count. This is a synthetic form of a natural hormone which helps your bone marrow recover and increases your white blood cell count after it has been lowered with chemotherapy. G-CSF is given as an injection under the skin (subcutaneously), similar to an insulin injection, either by the patient or a nurse every day for 3 to 14 days.

Anemia

The amount of red blood cells in the blood stream may also be affected by chemotherapy, but it does not usually drop too much.

Anemia may cause you to feel tired, dizzy, short of breath or chilly, so if you notice any of these symptoms you should report them to your doctor. Although you should eat well, anemia caused by chemotherapy is not usually helped by taking iron or B vitamins since the low red cell count is not caused by nutritional deficiencies but by a decreased production of red cells. If your anemia becomes severe enough to cause symptoms, your doctor may recommend a blood transfusion or, rarely, an injection of a hormone called 'erythropoeitin' (Epo®, Epogen®) which may help stimulate your bone marrow to make more red blood cells.

Abnormal bleeding or bruising

Platelets help to clot the blood. Chemotherapy may cause a temporary decrease of the platelet count. If this is severe enough, you may bleed easily. It is rare for low platelet counts to be a significant problem, but if you notice any abnormal bleeding or bruising you should report it to your doctor. ASA (Aspirin®) or

ASA-like drugs can slow down platelet function and should be taken only after checking with your doctor. However, acetaminophen (Tylenol®) does not affect the platelets and is generally all right to take in moderation.

Nausea and vomiting

Most of the chemotherapeutic drugs can cause nausea and vomiting, although some people are affected more than others. 'Antiemetic' drugs, which prevent nausea and vomiting, are usually given before the chemotherapy and every few hours afterwards for the first 24 to 48 hours. The nausea may start six to eight hours after the chemotherapy injection, or even the next day, and is usually not a prolonged problem. Eat something before the chemotherapy and regularly thereafter because it is often better not to have an empty stomach.

The nausea may feel like morning sickness, so it is sometimes helpful to take an antiemetic, have something to eat (for instance some dry crackers) and stay in bed for an hour to prevent vomiting. Avoid odors that cause more nausea. If the drugs you are given are not effective, tell your doctor so that different or additional antiemetics can be tried.

The drugs used to prevent nausea and vomiting include ondansetron (Zofran®), prochlorperazine (Stemetil®), dimenhydrinate (Gravol®), metoclopramide (Maxeran®, Nabilone®), and dexamethasone (Decadron®). Diphenhydramine (Benadryl®) and lorazepam (Ativan®) may also be helpful. Note that these drugs may also have side effects. For example, ondansetron (Zofran®) may cause headaches and constipation and prochlorperazine (Stemetil®) may cause restlessness that may require yet another drug, diphenhydramine (Benadryl®), for relief. The drugs may be given as pills, intravenous or intramuscular medications or rectal suppositories. The suppositories may be the easiest to take if you are vomiting or nauseated.

Some people also complain about stomach pain, an acidy feeling, heartburn, and a change in the taste in their mouth. These symptoms may be eased by food or antacids, but if the symptoms are severe, particularly the pain, you should notify your doctor.

Diarrhea and constipation

The anti-cancer drugs often cause some change in your bowel habits so don't be alarmed by minor disruptions. If you have severe diarrhea for more than 24 hours, or cramps, you should call your doctor because an anti-diarrheal drug may stop the problem. As well, you should be assessed to make sure this was actually related to the chemotherapy and not something totally unrelated. If you have diarrhea, try to drink lots of clear liquids to replace the fluid that you have lost and to rest your bowels. Avoid foods such as cabbage, beans, brans and spicy foods that cause loose bowels, gas, and cramps. Milk products may also contribute to diarrhea.

Some chemotherapy drugs may cause constipation. Often this can be avoided by drinking plenty of fluids, keeping active and possibly taking a mild stool softener. If you have a severe problem, notify your doctor.

Sore mouth (mucositis)

Many of the chemotherapy drugs cause soreness or dryness of the mouth and throat that can appear about five days after treatment begins. If this is a problem, avoid foods that irritate your mouth such as acidic, spicy or rough foods. Rinse your mouth often with baking soda and water. If your mouth gets so sore that you cannot eat, notify your doctor, as there are mouthwashes and painkillers that may ease your discomfort. People who tend to get cold sores (herpes) in addition to other mouth sores can be helped by an antiviral medication. If a white, cakey covering develops in your mouth you may have a yeast infection (candida) which may cause mouth soreness and difficulty eating and swallowing. A special mouthwash or pill may help.

Menstrual periods and sexuality

Chemotherapy may disrupt your menstrual periods, causing them to be irregular, to stop temporarily during chemotherapy and then return, or to stop permanently. This is not predictable, but it is more likely to happen in women closer to menopause than in younger women or if you are taking six months of chemotherapy rather than three months (see Menopause, below). If you are having menstrual changes, discuss them with your oncologist.

Chemotherapy drugs generally do not affect the ability to have sex, although you may notice changes. The mucosal lining of the vagina may feel dry or sore and it may be helpful to use a vaginal lubricant such as Replens®. As well, you may be at risk of getting a yeast (candida) infection which may irritate the area and may require treatment with antifungal creams. You may need to avoid certain sexual positions because of discomfort to your arm or chest area after surgery. Your libido, or sexual desire, may be affected by the stress of the illness, fatigue, your anxiety and the changes in your body which may affect your hormones, self-confidence and your body image. These are natural and normal responses that may be temporary. If you have continued difficulties with your sexual interest or activity, you and possibly your partner may want to discuss strategies to rekindle your sexuality with a professional counselor.

Menopause

Menopause is simply when menstrual periods stop completely. We now know that the hormonal changes that occur with menopause normally develop over a decade or so. At menopause the ovaries stop releasing eggs and make less estrogen. This decrease in the level of estrogen causes changes in the body in a wide variety of organs and tissues. In some women these changes are subtle and do not cause any problems. In other women they are troublesome and cause upsetting and frustrating symptoms.

Chemotherapy can bring on an early and abrupt menopause in some women due to the effect of the drugs on the ovaries. This is more common in women over the age of 40 and may depend on which drugs are used and the total doses prescribed. In some women the periods stop temporarily; in others they stop permanently. Even with blood tests and symptoms, it is sometimes difficult to know how complete the menopause is for six months to one year. The symptoms of menopause are often the most distressing part of the cancer treatment.

Menopause is a natural occurrence. It can be associated with the following symptoms and changes:

- dry skin
- dryness of the vagina and perineum
- hot flashes
- weight gain
- mood changes
- increase risk of osteoporosis (thin bones, decrease in the calcium content of the bones. Is called osteopenia when it is mild and osteoporosis when more severe. May be associated with an increased risk of bone fractures)
- increased risk of heart disease
- memory changes
- changes in libido.

Menopause is not the same for all women. It is important to have a discussion with your doctor about the symptoms you are having in context with your family history. If women in your family have a significant history of developing heart disease or osteoporosis at a young age, there may be specific precautions that you should start early. As well, your doctor may want to assess your bones with a bone density test. This test is like a bone scan but shows whether there is evidence of osteopenia or osteoporosis. Remember that you must assess your own symptoms and tailor recommendations according to what you are experiencing and your risks and your life style.

To avoid some of the problems associated with menopause:

- Stop smoking. It can cause heart disease, osteoporosis, lung disease and cancer.
- Do some exercise. Weight-bearing exercise can protect against osteoporosis; cardiopulmonary exercise is important for your heart and weight.
- Check your diet. Ensure that you have 1500 to 2000 mg of calcium in your diet or as supplements, 300 IU of vitamin D, and a low-fat, low-cholesterol diet.
- For vaginal dryness: a water-soluble lubricating jelly (e.g. Replens®) can help and make intercourse less painful. Occasionally, estrogen creams may be used sparingly.
- If you have hot flashes, limit your intake of caffeine, alcohol, chocolate, cola and stress, as they may exacerbate

hot flashes. Hot flashes may also be decreased with vitamin E, evening primrose oil, Remifemin® (black cohosh) or other herbal remedies. Other drugs that may help but require a prescription include Dixarit®, Bellagral®, Megace® and other progestins. The use of estrogen and progesterone for women with a history of breast cancer remains controversial but is being studied to assess the safety.

- Osteoporosis may be treated with medications such as biphosphonate (etidronate, clodrinate, Fosamax®) which decrease the bone changes and occasionally with progesterones and estrogens. New agents such as raloxifene are being licensed. Preliminary studies suggest it may protect against osteoporosis, heart disease, and possibly breast cancer.
- For changes in libido: It may just take time to get used to your body's changes. Occasionally, testosterone is recommended, as it may help encourage your sexual interest.

Discuss your symptoms and concerns with your doctor. It is important to remember that there is not one solution for all women. Menopausal changes and concerns and changes are very variable.

Prevent pregnancy during chemotherapy, but not with 'the pill'

Taking chemotherapy does not necessarily prevent pregnancy. Furthermore, IT IS IMPORTANT NOT TO GET PREGNANT WHILE ON CHEMOTHERAPY because these drugs, especially during the first three months of pregnancy, may cause damage and deformity of the fetus. While on chemotherapy, it is important to continue to use birth control measures; these should be discussed with your doctor. As your periods may be irregular, it may be difficult to predict the time of ovulation, so a combination of a barrier method (a condom or diaphragm) plus a spermicidal foam or gel is safest. Oral contraceptives are generally NOT recommended if you have breast cancer because estrogens are believed to stimulate some cancers.

Many women ask about having a baby after they have finished chemotherapy. If you continue to have periods and ovulate you may be able to get pregnant, but you should wait until you are fully recovered from the treatment and until you and your oncologist have discussed the risk of the cancer coming back. Pregnancy itself will not cause the cancer to come back, but the unpredictable nature of breast cancer and its potential for recurrence needs to be considered prior to a pregnancy.

General symptoms

All of the drugs may cause skin changes such as dryness, spots, increased sun sensitivity, or rashes. If you're going out in the sun wear protective clothing, including a sun hat. Many women complain about dry, gritty eyes which can be eased by eye drops or artificial tears. Other women complain of a flu-like feeling or of feeling cold for one to three days after the chemotherapy starts.

If the drug contains a dye (for example Adriamycin®, which is red) your urine may change color the day after you start chemotherapy as you excrete the drug. You do not need to take special precautions in the bathroom, as the chemotherapy drugs are not dangerous to anyone else: it is not like being radioactive! You should drink plenty of fluids to ensure a good urine flow and to prevent bladder irritation.

Some women develop joint or muscle aches and pains. These often begin after the chemotherapy is finished and can last several months. Fortunately, they are usually temporary and can be relieved with exercise or anti-inflammatory medications.

Certain drugs may cause tingling in the fingers and toes, and some people report a loss of muscle strength and a change in their sense of balance. This also should be temporary: if it is not, or if it interferes with your activities, report it to your doctor.

Some women complain of 'chemo brain,' claiming a loss in their short-term memory. This is often temporary and it is difficult to know if it is due to the chemotherapy, the stress of the illness or all the anti-nausea and other medications that are prescribed.

Other rare side effects may also occur, so if you experience a new problem that is unexpected you should report it to your doctor, as it may or may not be related to the chemotherapy. If you have finished your treatments and are on follow-up, you should probably report it to your family doctor, since your complaints may be unrelated to the therapy.

Other considerations while taking chemotherapy

While you are on chemotherapy you can eat whatever you like. However, if you are taking some other medication for another condition, your doctor should verify that it may be continued. Although some physicians and nutritionists recommend total abstinence from alcohol, an occasional glass of wine or beer is usually OK, but check with your doctor.

Fatigue levels vary. Some women are able to continue their normal activities and continue working throughout the chemotherapy. Others find the chemotherapy so physically or emotionally draining they need to take a leave from work. Although it is recommended that you remain as active as you can while on chemotherapy, you will need some extra rest. Since it's hard to predict how much rest you will need, it may be worthwhile to sit down with your family or your employer and warn them that there may be low-energy days.

Physical activity is important. If you exercise regularly you may want to continue, but tone down your routine to avoid straining yourself. Walks may replace your daily jogs.

Hormone Therapy

CHAPTER THIRTY

Hormone therapy: What is it and who benefits from it?

Hormones and hormone therapy

What are female hormones?

THE FEMALE HORMONES, estrogen and progesterone, control many of the female- and sex-related processes of the body, such as growth of female genitals and breasts, development of the female body shape and regulation of the menstrual cycle.

What is the relationship between hormones and breast cancer?

Estrogen not only stimulates the growth of the breasts, but it also appears to encourage the growth of some, but not all, breast tumors.

What is hormone therapy?

Hormone therapy for breast cancer is a form of whole-body (systemic) treatment that is used as adjuvant therapy or as treatment for cancer recurrence. The term 'hormone therapy' refers to a number of different treatments designed to reduce the level of female hormones in the body. These include the use of drugs, surgical removal of the ovaries (the ovaries produce estrogen in premenopausal women), or destruction of the ovaries by radiation (ablation of the ovaries). Hormone treatment is systemic because it affects hormone levels in the entire body. Changing the hormone levels affects the cancer cells and slows their growth. Hormone therapy may also be referred to as 'anti-estrogen therapy.' The most widely used and tested anti-estrogen drug is tamoxifen (Novaldex®, Tamofen®, etc.). Since this is the initial form of hormone therapy that most women take, this chapter will discuss the recommendations for this drug in detail.

Who should receive adjuvant tamoxifen?

As always, before deciding on any type of adjuvant therapy, the woman with breast cancer must be assessed to estimate her chances of the cancer recurring. The stage of the cancer must be reviewed (Chapter 17), taking into account the size of the cancer, the presence of cancer-involved lymph nodes, and the finding of lymphatic, vascular or neural cancerous invasion in the breast. Table 10 shows the assessment of cancer broadly categorized as low, moderate and high risk of recurrence, with the recommendations for or against adjuvant tamoxifen therapy in each category.

It is important to realize that these risk categories are useful, but are just general guidelines. Each woman's case is different and her risk of recurrence must be assessed based on other details in the pathology report in addition to these features. Therefore, a woman's risk may fit one of these categories exactly or be somewhere in between.

Tamoxifen works best in older women

With tamoxifen, the age of the woman is important: studies show that hormone therapy may be more beneficial to post-menopausal women than premenopausal women.

'ER-positive' or 'ER-negative'? Which type of tumor does tamoxifen attack best?

The pathologist can test a piece of the tumor using a chemical test to estimate how well the cancer is likely to respond to the anti-estrogen drug. This is done by measuring the amount of

Table 10 **Recommendations for the use of adjuvant tamoxifen**		
Low risk of recurrence	**Moderate risk of recurrence**	**High risk of recurrence**
All of:	Any *one* of:	Any *one* of:
Tumor less than 1 cm	Tumor more than 2 cm	Tumor more than 5 cm with cancerous lymph nodes
plus	**and/or**	**and/or**
No cancer in lymph nodes	1 to 7 lymph nodes with cancer	More than 8 lymph nodes with cancer
plus	**and/or**	**and/or**
No invasion into lymph channels, blood vessels of the breast, or into lymph nodes	Some invasion into lymph channels, blood vessels of the breast, or into lymph nodes	Skin invasion Chest wall invasion Inflammatory cancer
Recommendations for postmenopausal women		
No adjuvant tamoxifen	Adjuvant tamoxifen If ER-positive: tamoxifen with or without chemotherapy If ER-negative: chemotherapy plus tamoxifen	Intensive chemotherapy plus tamoxifen
Recommendations for premenopausal women		
No adjuvant therapy	Chemotherapy* (see Table 9) If ER-positive and tumor 1-2 cm and grade 1 or 2, tamoxifen may be recommended If ER-negative: no tamoxifen	Intensive chemotherapy plus tamoxifen

ER = estrogen receptor; see text
*Studies are being done of the addition of tamoxifen to chemotherapy.

'estrogen receptors' (ER) on the cancer cell. (The estrogen receptors are where the estrogen attaches to the tumor. The anti-estrogen drug interferes with the receptor, preventing the estrogen from 'landing' on the tumor.)

In general, the higher the estrogen receptor level, the more responsive the tumor will be to tamoxifen. If the pathologist measures low levels of estrogen receptors (less than 10 to 15 units), then this means that the tumor is not being affected very much by the estrogen in the body to begin with, so anti-estrogen therapy may not have as much benefit in these patients.

Most laboratories test estrogen receptor content of a cancer by 'immunoperoxidase staining.' With this test, the ER content of the tumor is reported as 0, +1, +2, or +3, with 0 representing virtually no estrogen receptor content and +3 a high ER content.

Other questions about tamoxifen

What is the dose?

Tamoxifen is usually taken daily as a single 20 mg dose or as a 10 mg dose twice a day. Today, most centers recommend continuing tamoxifen treatment for five years. There is currently no evidence of benefit from longer treatment.

Why don't postmenopausal women at low risk of cancer recurrence take tamoxifen?

Tamoxifen, like other therapy, does have some side effects that need to be considered and, at present, this group has not yet been proven to benefit sufficiently from the drug to warrant the small but real risk of side effects. This may change, however, as new studies of tamoxifen are completed.

Is tamoxifen only for postmenopausal women?

The beneficial effect of tamoxifen has been shown in many studies in postmenopausal women. Studies in premenopausal women suggest some benefit, but it may not be as great. Ongoing trials are looking at this question.

Does tamoxifen have other beneficial effects?

At menopause, women's chances of getting heart disease begin to increase. Tamoxifen seems to protect postmenopausal women from this increased risk of heart attacks by maintaining cholesterol and lipids at levels similar to those of premenopausal women. It also slows the loss of calcium from the bones and may reduce the chance of osteoporosis. However, protection from heart disease or osteoporosis is not a sufficient reason to recommend adjuvant tamoxifen therapy.

CHAPTER THIRTY-ONE

Side effects of hormone therapy

Do hormone therapies have side effects?

As with all other drug treatments, there are potential side effects associated with hormone treatments. These must be carefully discussed and considered before starting treatment. The side effects may depend on the dose or length of treatment.

Tamoxifen

Tamoxifen is an estrogen as well as an anti-estrogen. This means that it acts like an estrogen on some normal tissues, but blocks the estrogen receptors of the cancer cells.

Many women have no side effects from tamoxifen. Others notice some side effects, several of which are listed below.

Hot flashes are more pronounced in pre- and perimenopausal women and are often temporary.

Vaginal discharge: this may be clear or whitish. If you have a bloody discharge it is abnormal and should be investigated by your physician.

Weight gain is common but is usually only a few pounds.

Facial hair: this is not common and is usually very sparse.

Phlebitis: this is an inflamed vein that contains a blood clot. It occurs in about 1% of women taking tamoxifen for five years. It is dangerous because the clot can dislodge and travel to other parts of the body, especially the lungs, causing a pulmonary embolus (blockage of a blood vessel at the lungs). Phlebitis and blood clots are more frequent in women who are also getting chemotherapy at the same time as the tamoxifen, in women with a previous history of phlebitis, and in women who have other risk factors such as a history of smoking. If you have a swollen or painful leg or calf muscle, see your doctor. If the diagnosis confirms a blood clot, medication may be prescribed to dissolve the clot and tamoxifen should probably be stopped.

Continuation of menstruation: for premenopausal women, ovulation and menses may continue so birth control precautions should be maintained. The drug's effect on a fetus is not known.

Nausea or vomiting, loss of appetite: these are rare and usually temporary.

Rash, skin dryness and hair loss: these are very rare.

Headache, depression and dizziness: also rare.

Fatigue and malaise: rare.

Hypercalcemia (high calcium levels in the blood): this usually occurs only if there are bone metastases. If you get very thirsty, constipated, nauseated and confused, your blood calcium level should be checked.

Flare-up of pain: metastatic cancer may react to the tamoxifen by becoming more painful. This is called a 'flare reaction' and is usually temporary. It is considered to be a good sign, indicating that the cancer is responding to the tamoxifen.

Endometrial (uterine) cancer: some women taking tamoxifen have been found to develop cancer of the endometrium. At the currently recommended dose of 20 mg per day for five years, approximately two women per 1,000 will develop endometrial cancer each year. This is two to three times higher than the risk in the general population of women not taking tamoxifen. For women with invasive breast cancers larger than 1 cm, the chance of developing endometrial cancer while taking tamoxifen is less than the benefit of avoiding a recurrence of breast cancer by taking tamoxifen. However, if you have any unexplained vaginal bleeding you should see your doctor. As well, you should have an annual pelvic examination.

Retinal changes: very rare. Vision changes from tamoxifen have very rarely been reported. If you notice a change in your sight you should see an ophthalmologist (eye doctor).

Liver tumors: these have occurred in women taking tamoxifen but are very rare and may be benign.

Other anti-estrogens

New anti-estrogens are being developed that act in a similar way as tamoxifen but may have different side effects. For example, droloxifene, raloxifene,
toremifene and trioxifene have been shown to have some effect on breast cancer and are being tested to assess their side effects and potential usefulness. Pure antiestrogens (e.g. Faslodex®) are also being tested to see if they have advantages over tamoxifen, both in terms of decreased side effects and increased effectiveness.

Progestins (e.g. megestrol acetate [Megace®])

Although megestrol acetate is commonly used, it is not entirely clear how it works. However, this and other progestins have been shown to be effective in treating metastatic breast cancer, with an overall response rate of about 28%. Megestrol and high-dose medroxyprogesterone acetate have been shown to be as effective as tamoxifen.

Megace® is well tolerated. The following side effects may occur.

Weight gain, the major side effect, occurs in 20% to 50% of patients. The weight gain may be only a few pounds or may be more, and is related to the dose of the drug. The higher the dose the more frequent and greater the weight gain. Both an increase in appetite and fluid retention are responsible for the extra pounds.

Vaginal bleeding occurs in 5% to 10% of women. It sometimes happens while taking the drug but occurs more often when it is discontinued. A vaginal discharge may also occur.

Hot flashes are much less common than with tamoxifen, but may occur.

High blood pressure is rare.

High blood sugar level: patients with diabetes who already have elevated blood sugars may need to adjust their diabetes medication if the sugars get too high due to the megestrol.

Nausea and vomiting have been reported in about 10% of women on megestrol.

Headaches and depression may occur infrequently.

Rash and itch have been reported.

Increased level of calcium is rare but can occur in women with bone metastases.

Rarely, a mild decrease in the white blood cell count and/or platelet counts have been reported.

Fluid retention, which is usually mild.

Other progestins such as medroxyprogesterone acetate may cause an increase in acne or facial hair, constipation, muscle cramps, skin abscesses, increased sweating, mild fatigue, and congestive heart failure as well as the same side effects as megestrol. Hair loss has also been reported.

Aromatase inhibitors

Aromatase inhibitors are a group of drugs that block an enzyme that makes estrogen in the body and in the tumor. These are effective in postmenopausal women. Anastrozole (Arimidex®) and letrozole (Femara®) have recently been licensed and have replaced an older medication named aminoglutethimide (Cytadren®). Both drugs have been studied in clinical trials and have been shown to be both active and safe. The side effects of both drugs are similar and quite rare. These are listed below.

Hot flashes may be worse the first month or two. Avoiding caffeine, alcohol, chocolate and stress may be helpful.

Headache is usually mild.

Nausea may be worse the first two weeks or so and then usually disappears.

Swelling/edema is rare and usually mild.

Weight gain: rare.

Since anastrozole and letrozole are new drugs, other side effects may eventually be added to this list.

Androgens

Androgens are male hormones that can be used to treat metastatic breast cancer. Fluoxymesterone (Halotesin®) has been commonly used and is effective. There are a number of side effects.

A masculinizing effect may include scalp hair loss, growth of facial hair, lowering of the voice, increase in size of the clitoris and increase in body hair. The extent of the side effects depends on the dose, the duration of treatment and the individual. These effects may not completely reverse when the drug is stopped.

Weight gain is usually mild.

Nausea and decreased appetite may occur occasionally, and even less so with low doses of the drug.

Inhibitors of the pituitary hormones

The pituitary gland makes a number of hormones that control specific glands such as the ovary. Several drugs have been used to try to decrease the levels of these 'controlling' hormones. The most promising are medications that interfere with FSH (follicular stimulating hormone) and LH (luteinizing hormone), hormones that control the ovaries. Without FSH and LH the ovary stops making many of the estrogens. Studies are being done with drugs that consist of a combination of tamox-

What can be done about side effects?

Listing all of the side effects of these drugs is depressing. The thing to remember is that most women do not experience many of these side effects. The positive side, of course, is that the drugs are being given because of their beneficial anti-cancer effects. Each woman should evaluate the risks and benefits of treatment on an individual basis with her doctors.

If you experience any side effects it is important to discuss them with your doctors and nurses, since they may be able to offer helpful suggestions or remedies. The three commonest side effects of hormone therapy are mild nausea, hot flashes and vaginal dryness/irritation. The nausea often goes away after two to three weeks. Some practical tips regarding control of mild nausea and decreased appetite are described in Chapter 36; more severe nausea and vomiting are usually treated with drugs.

Hot flashes can sometimes be reduced in severity or frequency by avoiding caffeine, alcohol and stress or by altering the time of day that you take your medication. Some drugs can be taken in a divided dose which may reduce hot flashes (for example, take tamoxifen in doses of 10 mg twice a day instead of 20 mg at night). Low-dose clonidine (Dixarit®), a prescription medication, may help reduce the hot flashes. Many women have developed 'home remedies' which seem to work for them and, although not proven, vitamin E (800 I.U. daily), evening primrose oil, and Remifemin®, among others, have been helpful. Soy products may also be helpful.

Vaginal dryness and irritation can make intercourse uncomfortable or impossible. A water-soluble lubricating jelly (for example, K-Y®, Replens® or Muko®; available in your drugstore) may be helpful. This jelly should be applied to the vaginal opening and to the head of the penis to make initiation of intercourse easier. Petroleum-based jellies (i.e. Vaseline) are not advised since they are messy and get sticky with rubbing, making matters worse. If symptoms are very severe and the above is unsuccessful, occasionally it is helpful to use a small amount of estrogen vaginal cream applied to the opening of the vagina daily for two weeks (not injected into the vagina as usually recommended) and then about once per week. Some of the estrogen may be absorbed into the blood stream, but one has to balance quality of life against any small potential risk due to the estrogen.

ifen and these inhibitors of pituitary hormones, for example, leuprolide (Lupron®) and goserelin (Zoladex®). These drugs have very few side effects. Menstrual periods will stop in pre-menopausal women but this may take three to four months. Hot flashes and other menopausal symptoms may occur but will stop when the drug is discontinued. Rare instances of nausea, depression, increased bone pain, and swelling of the eyelids or breasts have also been reported.

PART THREE | **Beyond the initial phase of treatment**

Coping with Cancer

CHAPTER THIRTY-TWO

Living with a diagnosis of breast cancer

by Carolyn Baker, RN

ALTHOUGH EVERY PERSON with cancer and every family member is unique, the road each must travel is well worn by the millions of others who have come before. It is a journey marked by hope and despair, courage and fear, humor and anger, and constant uncertainty. While the body undergoes tests and treatments, the mind searches for its own way of coping. This section is dedicated to the emotional effects of the diagnosis and treatment of cancer — the side of cancer that neither surgery nor chemotherapy nor radiation can treat.

Is there a 'right way' to feel after receiving a cancer diagnosis?

Many women are concerned that the thoughts and feelings that they experience following a diagnosis of cancer are somehow abnormal or crazy and that there must be a 'right way' to feel. This couldn't be further from the truth. There is no one way to feel. Reactions to the diagnosis can span the full range of human emotion: anger, anxiety, uncertainty, hopelessness, helplessness, depression, a feeling of isolation, vulnerability, relief that there really is something wrong, and even guilt that one has somehow contributed to the development of her own disease, or delayed in bringing it to a doctor's attention.

It is important to realize that the initial reaction to the diagnosis will be followed by other feelings. Just as we go through a series of 'stages' in accepting the loss of a loved one, we pass through a number of emotional levels on our way to acknowledging the diagnosis of cancer. First, there is often disbelief in the diagnosis, denial that it is true, and anger at being 'singled out.' Finally, there is usually an acknowledgement that 'Yes, I do have cancer.' Why we go through these stages is difficult to know. Psychologists postulate that the time required to progress from disbelief to acknowledgement may offer protection by creating time and space for adjustment.

> 'I felt shocked...numb...like it wasn't real. I don't think I really felt anything for a week and then I felt betrayed.'
>
> 'I decided that the doctors had made a mistake and that any minute someone would come out and say it had all been an unfortunate mistake.'

Denial is often a prominent response early in the cancer experience. It is a defense against fear and helps to maintain emotional equilibrium. It is not uncommon to hear people comment, 'I think she's in denial,' as if there may be something unusual and potentially dangerous about this reaction. In fact, some degree of denial is normal and is probably necessary to protect oneself and to maintain the hope needed to participate in daily life. However, it is important to recognize that denial is healthy only as long as it does not interfere with seeking medical care or participating in appropriate treatment.

> 'At some level I had to distance myself from the reality of the cancer in order to listen to the information that I was being given. I had to think that this was about someone else...It really protected me but it drove my husband crazy.'

Expressions of very strong emotion are to be expected and they may range from anger and bitterness to frank hostility which may be directed at anyone and anything.

'I was angry at everyone...God in particular... I hadn't done anything to deserve this.'

'I was furious. I really didn't think that I needed to get cancer in order to be better at my job or to be a better person. Someone was playing a cruel joke.'

Fortunately, most people will emerge from the storm of emotions to reach a point of equilibrium and acknowledgement, although it is common to move back and forth from one 'stage' to another. Many think about having cancer in the past tense. This helps the woman to keep the cancer from dominating her life and allows her to remain more positive, even if she is well aware of the possibility of recurrence.

'Have I accepted my diagnosis of cancer? I don't know. After six months I still often wish it wasn't so, think that it isn't so and remember that it is. It's a constant back-and-forth.'

Coping with cancer

Every person has a unique tool box of coping strategies that we add to over a lifetime. Most will find what they need to meet the challenge of cancer.

'How did I cope initially? I don't know, really... I guess I did the things that I've done in other tough situations...I turned to my family and friends, then the nurses and doctors.'

There are as many coping skills as there are people. Seeking information, turning to family, friends and others in a similar situation for support, developing a partnership with the health care team, maintaining hope, and learning stress management techniques are all means by which the coping 'mindset' develops.

Seeking information

Appropriate information can help to allay much of the anxiety and fear associated with the unknown. The type and amount required varies with the wants and needs of the woman and her family. Generally, people want to know about diagnostic tests, treatment plan (purpose, expected results, side effects, length of time and scheduling), and prognosis. Essential but often neglected information concerns how the disease and treatment are likely to affect the person's daily life. Your cancer center in your local chapter of the Cancer Society may provide this kind of help. There are booklets, seminars, stress management training, and self-help groups for individuals with cancer and their families.

Of course, the health care team is a critical provider of information pertinent to your particular problem. When attending appointments with members of the health care team, don't be afraid to ask questions. They will be expecting it. Prepare a list; otherwise, you may forget important points that you have been wondering about. Write down the answers and, if you wish, take someone along to help you remember what was said. The early phase of diagnosis and treatment can be somewhat of a daze and having a spare pair of ears around is very helpful.

Telling others

In most cases, your family and close friends will learn sooner or later that you have cancer. It is usually best to disclose the information yourself, according to your own schedule. Confiding fears and hopes is an important part of developing the coping mindset, and in the long run it is easier than trying to conceal these important feelings.

There are some situations in which it may be best not to tell. Family members who are too old, too young, or too emotionally fragile may have difficulty accepting or understanding the situation. However, it is quite extraordinary how most people can summon the courage to adapt to the reality of a potentially life-threatening illness, even when it involves someone whom they love very much.

Sometimes family members are the first to learn the diagnosis and they will occasionally attempt to shield the person with cancer from the information in what is usually a misguided but well meant attempt to protect her from the pain of knowing. In certain instances, such as when the woman is extremely old or very ill and cannot understand, this is sensible. In the vast majority of cases, however, it is better, and her right, for her to know. Important relationships that should be strengthened can become strained and artificial as loving family members and friends try to skirt the issue and discuss only superficial matters. Worse than that, in almost all such cases, the woman finds out anyway, all too often at an inopportune and harmful moment.

Women usually have a lot of anxiety about how best to explain to their children about the cancer when they are trying to cope, themselves, with what it all means. They are worried about being able to care for their children during treatment, and whether they will be around to help them grow up. The goal in telling children is to give them opportunities to ask questions about the disease and to express their feelings about it. While we all wish to shield our children from 'bad news,' it is better that they experience pain in a way that they understand and can talk about with their parents than to cope with sorrow on their own in forms that become embellished by their imagination. Moreover, if they are denied knowledge of the cause of why there has been great disruption in the family, they may become confused and hurt and mistakenly believe that they are responsible. There are several excellent books available which can help you to explain 'cancer' to children of various ages (see Additional Reading). As well, there may be support groups for children such as art therapy sessions.

Support groups

In most cities and towns there are support groups consisting of people with cancer and trained professionals who manage the sessions. The professionals provide a forum where the person with cancer can be open about her thoughts and feelings, and can discover that these are normal and acceptable. Other members of the group often suggest alternative ways to deal with difficult issues, ways that have helped them. Seeing others who are coping with similar situations can aid in identifying solutions to problems which seem overwhelming initially. In addition, membership in a formal group may give the person with cancer the means to overcome a feeling of helplessness by offering assistance to others.

'Although my family was supportive, I felt as if they couldn't possibly understand what it was like for me. I needed to talk to someone else who had cancer. That doesn't mean that you shouldn't talk to your family but it's different when you talk to another survivor. In the Living with Cancer Group, I found that I could give something back...which was very important as it was the first time in a long time that I felt useful.'

Breast Cancer Visitors

As well as formal support groups, most women will benefit from meeting with a 'survivor.' The Breast Cancer Visitors program of the Cancer Society is an invaluable resource to the woman with a new diagnosis of breast cancer. Ideally, this contact should occur while the woman is considering surgery or still in hospital.

As these women have 'been there,' they provide women with information about living with breast cancer — from talking to family and friends, to buying a bathing suit with suitable support. They also provide a 'shoulder to cry on.'

You do not need to wait for a referral from a doctor or nurse to initiate a Breast Cancer Visitors visit. Any woman (or her family and friends) can call the Cancer Society to request a visit either before surgery, during the hospital stay, or afterwards.

'When the volunteer walked through the door and said that she was ten years out from diagnosis, I felt an enormous weight melt away. She gave me more hope with her presence than anyone else had with their words.'

Developing a partnership with the health care team

At one time, patients and families were considered to be silent members of the health care team, if indeed they were considered team members at all. Today, people with cancer are encouraged to take an active role in treatment planning.

The first step in developing a partnership with the health care team is to know who the players are and what each one has to offer. This can be a challenging task as, over time, there are often many different specialists involved in the care of the patient and family. It is important to identify one team member who will serve as the leader: often the family doctor, the oncologist (cancer specialist) or a specialist nurse. It doesn't matter who assumes the role as long as he or she is able to relate to the woman and her family and will be there for the duration. This person should be available at regular intervals, or when required, to listen to concerns, to direct questions to the appropriate professionals, and to serve as a guide and support.

The second important step is to participate in decision-making about treatment.

> 'I had a life-threatening illness and I was being asked whether I wanted this treatment or that treatment. I felt that my life was on the line if I made the wrong decision. I didn't know whether or not I wanted that responsibility. Then I realized that I knew me better than anyone else and that knowledge would be helpful in making a good decision.'

No matter how complex your problem may seem, your health care team members should be able to help you through the decision-making processes by providing you with the framework of the 'big picture,' thereby simplifying decisions. His or her ability to explain things is essential in providing you with the information you need to participate. Once a few of the initial choices are made based on such information, you will have some time to seek additional resources and pursue the educational process that will support you later on.

Participating in decision-making means listening to the options, identifying their advantages and disadvantages, and comparing them to your own values and aspirations and those of your family. Some women will want to discuss all of the options, perhaps seeking a second opinion before making an informed decision with or without their families. Others might be uncomfortable making the final decision, but can still participate by clarifying their values and wishes so that the final recommendations for treatment can be tailored to their needs.

The third step in developing a partnership with the health care team is to participate in the treatment plan — managing the side effects of the treatment, reporting changes in condition, attending follow-up appointments, providing team members with feedback about how things are progressing, and using the services and supports that are available.

A note about changing doctors

Clearly, excellent communication between each woman and her doctor is critically important to the successful adaptation to the diagnosis and treatment. Unfortunately, some physicians never learn to speak comfortably with their patients or families and in the name of some sort of professionalism let people down by not 'being there' for them when tough choices have to be made. Although such physicians may appear to be abrupt, aloof and uncaring, this is not usually the case. Nevertheless, if this problem creates a barrier, ask your family doctor to refer you to someone else. Remember, you almost always have a choice in who treats you, so don't be afraid to find someone who you are comfortable with. Keep in mind, however, that a decision to change physicians should be based on reality and not on a quest to find a doctor who will promise a cure and guarantee to relieve all your fears.

When friends don't call

Lost and strained friendships can be a particularly painful aspect of dealing with cancer. Friends may not call for a variety of reasons. For most, it is because they feel that they will have so little to say that will help, and they fear that instead they might say something hurtful. Others may be afraid that they will not be able to respond appropriately to your change of appearance, or they are fearful of facing the possibility of your death and the eventuality of their own.

> 'I see that my friends don't know how to talk to me, and they shy away from me.'

If you believe it is discomfort that is keeping a particular friend from visiting, you might try a phone call to dissolve the barrier. This often reassures them that you are still the same person that they liked before, and that you understand their difficulty. However, don't expect to change or enlighten everyone. We all have our own emotional capabilities and timetables and some people will not be comforted sufficiently for them to maintain the relationship as it was before. You will find that different friends will provide suppport in different ways at different times, and you will make new friends along the way who are participating in the same treatment process.

Sexuality

Sexuality need not be affected by the diagnosis of breast cancer but it often is. Many women feel mutilated by the surgery and uncomfortable with their bodies. Also, treatment can cause fatigue and other symptoms that decrease desire. In addition, the onset of treatment-induced menopause may make intercourse uncomfortable due to vaginal dryness.

The whole process of the diagnosis and treatment may make a woman less interested in sex. Her focus may be on other issues or she may feel depressed. This is normal and needs to be openly discussed with her partner. Her partner may also be frightened about losing and/or hurting her. A common myth is that cancer may be contagious. This is entirely false.

By recognizing these changes and seeking counselling if necessary, these feelings may improve with time and understanding. A satisfying sexual relationship is possible after breast cancer.

Maintaining hope

Hope is a crucial tool for people with cancer and their families. It is the internal resource that permits one to cope with the stresses associated with diagnosis and treatment. Loss of hope reduces one's ability to adjust to the situation.

Hope means different things to different people, and tends to change over time depending on the stage of the disease and treatment:

> 'There is always hope, it just changes. First you hope that you don't have cancer, then you hope that the cancer is curable or at least treatable. Then you hope for time and finally, you hope for a good going. If you lose hope you give up.'

Maintaining and nurturing hope is a strategy that can allay anxiety, depression and fear. Nurturing hope means focusing on the present and what is immediately ahead, rather than on the future or the past, neither of which can be changed. While this reorientation of focus can be difficult in our future-oriented society, it can help manage the daily challenges of cancer treatment.

Hope can be affected by the behavior of others. Family members and friends can support the idea that being hopeful is a good thing, and they should not classify hope as being false.

> 'Be prepared for the worst but hope for the best. There is no such thing as false hope. Every day I hope for a miracle, but that doesn't stop me from continuing my treatment nor would it stop me from acceptance if my treatment is no longer working. If you took my hope away I don't know if I would want to continue...'

Hope is not based on false optimism or benign reassurance, but is built on the belief that better days or moments can come in spite of the situation.

CHAPTER THIRTY-THREE

How can your family and friends help you cope with breast cancer?

by Maria Hugi, MD,
and members of the Treasure Chests support group

THIS CHAPTER IS BASED ON the wisdom of the women in Treasure Chests, a breast cancer support group in Vancouver. We have all had to face breast cancer and range in age from 30 to 75. All of us agree that the support that we have received from friends and family makes the day-to-day fight against breast cancer much easier to deal with.

Breaking the news

Friends and family members are often caught off guard by your diagnosis of breast cancer and don't know how to respond. One of our members recounted her friend's reaction to breast cancer:

> "When I called my friend and told her about my diagnosis, there was a long pause, a deep breath and then she said, 'OK, what do we do now?' I know that she was shocked and frightened for me, but her response told me that my breast cancer involved her too and that I could count on her to help."

Another member's husband told his wife, upon diagnosis, that he would do anything to change places with her, that he wished that he had the cancer. While you are reeling from the shock and uncertainty of the diagnosis, you need to feel that everyone is on your side and that everyone appreciates your fears.

Practical support

Practical help was very important to us during our breast cancer treatments. One member's colleagues organized a 'meals on wheels' for her during her radiation treatment to provide her with three meals a day. Another member recalled how her 75-year-old father got up twice a night to feed her 4-month-old son so that she could get a good night's sleep.

One woman felt that her friends and family would have done anything for her, but she often hesitated to ask. Don't hesitate to ask. Your friends and family are frantic with fear for you and feel so powerless to help you with the cancer that anything tangible they can do for you makes them feel better.

So ask friends or family members to take you to your chemotherapy and radiation treatments, and to your clinic appointments in order to be that extra set of ears. Ask them to bring over your favorite food. Get them to do the grocery shopping and the laundry. Let them clean the house, mow the lawn and look after the car. Get them to babysit the kids and help with child care. Accept their offer to take you to a humorous play or movie.

Have them go wig shopping with you. Get them to give you hats as gifts, instead of flowers. Of course, flowers are nice too, as are the occasional boxes of chocolates! One of our members needed help with her Christmas baking. Get your friends to help you with holiday preparations. During our treatments, a lot of us found it tedious to write Christmas cards or thank-you notes for gifts and flowers. Get your friends or relatives to help you write them.

The single women living alone in our group welcomed daily telephone calls from friends and family. These women also needed friends or family to spend nights with them at times, especially when they were feeling particularly ill or vulnerable. A daughter of one of our members moved back home to be with her mother during treatment. Another woman who lives alone recalled how, during treatment, she appreciated friends who looked after her cat.

Your friends and family can be of real help to you in getting information about breast cancer. In one case, a woman's sisters helped her greatly by calling the toll free 1-888-939-3333 Cancer Information Service and following up on the information. Another's husband read all that he could get his hands on about breast cancer at the cancer center's library. A cousin, who was a medical doctor, took time off work to attend breast cancer conferences at the cancer center. Still another's friend surfed the Internet for breast cancer information.

Let your friends and family filter through the information for you if you feel exhausted or overwhelmed. One of our members who is a medical doctor said that for the first two years after diagnosis she couldn't work up the courage to read anything about breast cancer because she took it all too personally. Fortunately, her physician husband constantly searched the medical literature for information.

Emotional support

All of us wanted to be listened to unconditionally, especially when we needed to rant and rave and feel sorry for ourselves. We appreciated friends and family members who were not afraid to talk about breast cancer. One woman felt that none of her friends or family members shared their feelings and fears regarding her illness with her. As a result, she spent a lot of time reassuring them that she would be fine.

Many of us wanted to be hugged, especially when the tears flowed. One young woman valued getting hugged by her male friends. It made her feel that her scarred body might still be attractive, and boosted her sense of femininity.

Everyone drew strength from frequent phone calls and visits. Some enjoyed going for walks with friends. One woman was touched to receive letters and cards from her friend, nieces and nephews telling her what a wonderful person she was to them.

Another woman, who chose not to have the recommended chemotherapy and radiation treatments, needed and received the support and encouragement from her friends to pursue alternative treatments.

Friends and relatives need to know when to leave you in peace. A group member who is retired remarked that the support sometimes became 'too much'; that she, and especially her husband, found the frequent visitors overwhelming. Some of us felt that we had to entertain our friends and relatives when they visited.

There were mixed feelings in our group about self-help books, motivational tapes, megavitamin diets or herbal remedies given to us, with the best of intentions, by friends and relatives. Some women really appreciated this type of advice and were able to muster up the energy to take it to heart. Others felt that this type of help made them feel guilty and that these gifts implied that they were somehow responsible for their disease.

Most of us were also leery of advice to think positively. In fact, some of us were almost moved to fisticuffs at the mention of the words. Again, we felt that there was an implication that if we had been positive thinkers, none of this would have happened. Relatives and friends have to bear in mind that it is extremely difficult to think positively, let alone get out of bed in the morning, when you're exhausted by your treatment.

Humor was something that most of us appreciated. One woman enjoyed friends making jokes about her bald head. Another was regularly faxed amusing cartoons and stories. Still others were given humorous books and videos.

Partners, sex and support

We all agreed that sex was probably the last thing on our minds during treatment. The insult that a woman's body receives from breast cancer, coupled with her treatment, wreaks havoc with her sex drive and sense of femininity. Most of us found it exhausting to even smear on some lipstick! Your partner has to understand that your treatment can throw you into early menopause and that you may be riding an emotional roller coaster while trying to come to terms with your disease.

Some of us with mastectomies felt, as women, that we were whole again when our partners touched our scarred chest. Other women felt awkward and said that they had difficulty touching the mastectomy area themselves for fear that they might detect a return of the cancer. It was important for us to feel loved by our partners and reassured that the loss of a breast did not make us less attractive to them.

Many of us worried that our partners weren't getting enough emotional support from our friends and family since it was us who were always everyone's center of concern. One woman felt sorry for her husband and wondered what he must be thinking when some acquaintances, insensitively, would tell 'boob' jokes within his earshot. He seemed to take it in stride. However, she was amazed at the number of breast jokes that he had to bear.

Our partners seemed to prefer to care for our practical needs but encouraged us to seek as much emotional support as we needed. Some said that they were extremely relieved when we attended a breast cancer support group. In fact, one husband found out about our support group for his wife. Another husband became quite agitated with his wife when she decided, for a trivial reason, not to attend the monthly support group meeting.

Vulnerable times

The weekend before your first treatments can be a very anxiety-riddled time for you. That's when your friends and family need to rally round and listen to your fears or help you with practical things around the house.

You may also have a difficult time when your breast cancer treatments come to an end. Suddenly, you will no longer be under the intense scrutiny of your health-care providers and you may feel somewhat abandoned. Your ongoing fears of the cancer returning may escalate at this time, especially since you are no longer actively fighting the disease with therapy. Your family and friends need to be aware of these fears so that they can support you. Breast cancer is a frightening disease that can undermine you on every front. However, sympathetic relatives and friends can help you in your fight against this disease or, as one of our members put it, 'help you get your life back.'

CHAPTER THIRTY-FOUR

Physical therapy and management of lymphedema
by Susan Harris, PhD, PT,
and Maria Hugi, MD

MANY OF THE BREAT CANCER treatments such as surgery, radiation and chemotherapy have side effects that can be minimized or eliminated by physical therapy. By working to prevent the physical limitations that can occur, physical therapists can help to restore and maintain your overall health and fitness, and enhance your quality of life.

What to do before treatments begin

Even before you begin your treatments for breast cancer, it is a good idea to consult a physical therapist who can take 'baseline' measurements of your shoulder motion, upper body strength, arm circumference and overall fitness level. These measurements will help both you and the physical therapist monitor your progress as you return to your pre-treatment levels of health and fitness.

At this pre-treatment visit, the physical therapist can instruct you in gentle exercises of the hand, wrist, elbow, and shoulder that you can do within a day or two after your surgery. She or he can also advise you about aerobic conditioning programs to improve your overall cardiovascular fitness while you are undergoing your treatments.

Exercising during and after breast cancer treatment

Most women with breast cancer have at least two types of surgery. One removes the tumor from the breast (lumpectomy, mastectomy) and the second type, axillary dissection, is done to determine whether the breast cancer has spread to the lymph nodes underneath the arm (see Chapter 19). It is the axillary dissection which leads to difficulties in shoulder motion and weakness, and which can contribute to later arm swelling.

After any type of surgery, one can expect some pain, discomfort, stiffness and swelling. This is especially true after axillary dissection. Up to 50% of women who undergo this procedure develop tightness, pain, and the formation of 'cords' in the armpit, inner elbow and wrist within a few weeks after their surgery. These thin, visible cords are the hardened lymphatic vessels which have been interrupted by the removal of axillary lymph nodes. Some degree of arm motion may be temporarily lost due to this cording, but within several weeks the cords will rupture on their own and arm motion will return. Physical therapy can help you return to your pre-surgical levels of shoulder motion and upper body strength.

During and after radiation therapy

During and after radiation therapy you may be tired and feel that exercise is the last thing in the world you want to do. However, the physical therapist can devise a helpful aerobic exercise program for you and recommend specific exercises to help regain shoulder motion and upper body strength that will help offset any stiffness in the chest and shoulder muscles that can occur due to radiation therapy.

During and after chemotherapy

Although you may feel tired during and after your chemotherapy, it is important not only to get extra rest but also to maintain your overall fitness level by exercising regularly, at least three to five days per week. Chemotherapy can also cause joint pain or stiffness similar to arthritis-like pains. Specific types of regular exercise that is gentle on your joints, such as walking or swimming or riding a stationary bicycle, may help during this period. Moist heat such as hot packs or a warm bath can help ease joint and muscle aches. Also, cold packs can help reduce acute (sudden) joint pain or swelling.

How can a physical therapist help during your recovery?

Physical therapists can help you regain or improve your range of shoulder motion, upper body strength, and aerobic or cardiovascular fitness. Also, they can teach you how to massage the scar tissue from your breast and axillary surgery. And finally, a physical therapist can measure and monitor the circumference of your arm for swelling that might be an early sign of lymphedema.

Range of shoulder motion

The most important problem to tackle is to regain full, pretreatment levels of shoulder motion. Although some women regain full motion within days after their surgery, many women have trouble. This is seen especially when trying to: 1) lift your arm forward and up over you head (shoulder flexion), 2) raise your arm out and up at the side (shoulder abduction), and 3) bring your arm behind your back to fasten a bra (shoulder internal rotation). The following exercises can help you regain these motions. We recommend that you do these exercises gently within the first week after surgery and progress to more active stretching by the second week.

The first two exercises should be done while lying on your back on the floor. In the first exercise (Figure 39), use a broomstick or cane to have the uninvolved arm 'help' stretch the involved arm into the final ranges of shoulder flexion. Stretch slowly, as far as you can comfortably go, exerting a prolonged pull on the affected arm. In the second floor exercise (Figure 40), put your hands underneath your head and slowly bring both elbows down to the floor. Breathe out as you stretch to try to get your elbows to touch the floor. Then relax and breathe in.

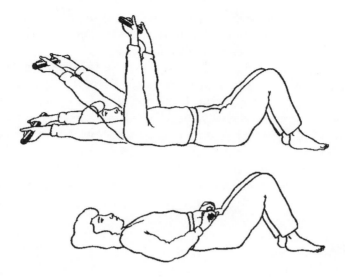

Figure 39: Holding a broomstick helps the unaffected arm stretch the affected arm in this exercise. (Figures 39 to 45 from *Recovering from breast surgery: exercises to strengthen your body and relieve pain.* Diane Stumm, Hunter House, 1995.)

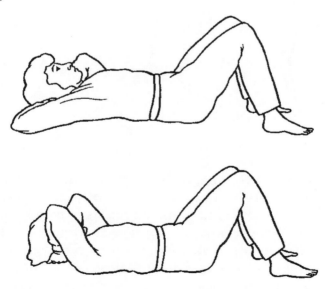

Figure 40: With hands behind your head, elbows are slowly brought down to the floor.

Breathe out again as you try to stretch a bit further. Repeat each of these exercises four to five times, making sure that your stretches are slow, steady and prolonged.

The third shoulder stretching exercise (Figure 41a) is performed while sitting in a chair or on the floor. It helps to do this exercise in front of a mirror. Once again, use a slow, steady and prolonged stretch to pull your affected arm up over your head and toward your ear. After each stretch, lower your arms and relax. Repeat the stretch four to five times. Once you can do this comfortably, you can increase the pull by bending your trunk sideways toward the side opposite to the involved arm (Figure 41b).

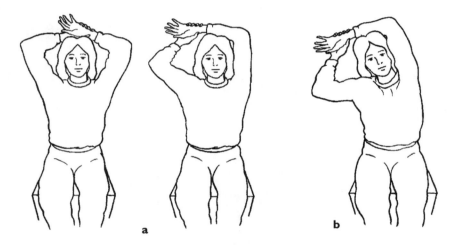

Figure 41: The affected arm is slowly and steadily stretched over your head.

The following two exercises will improve shoulder flexion. Stand facing a wall, with your feet about six inches away from the wall (Figure 42). Try to 'walk' the fingers of both hands up the wall while standing in place. When you have gone as high as you can comfortably go (while feeling a slow, prolonged stretch to your underarm muscles), hold that position for 5 to 10 seconds to maintain the stretch. To gauge your progress, put a pencil mark at the furthest point to which you can 'walk' your affected arm.

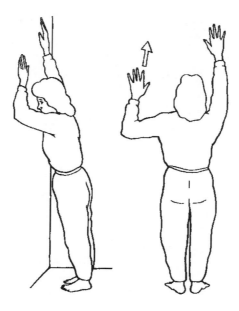

Figure 42: 'Walk' your fingers slowly up the wall, and then maintain the stretch for a few seconds.

Another shoulder flexion stretch (Figure 43) is done while you are on your hands and knees on the floor. With your hands directly underneath your shoulders and your knees about 10 to 12 inches apart, slowly lean back on your feet and lower your head to the floor. Keep your elbows straight and feel the pull in your underarm area. Hold the stretch for 5 to 10 seconds and then return to the hands-and-knees position. Repeat the stretch four to five times.

Strengthening exercises

It used to be said that vigorous exercises should not be done after breast and axillary surgery. This is no longer true. Once you have full shoulder range of motion, at four to eight weeks after surgery you can begin to add exercises to increase upper body strength. In the stretching exercise shown in Figure 39, for example, you can add a 1- to 2-pound (1/2- to 1-kg) weight in each hand and alternately stretch each arm up over your shoulder to strengthen the shoulder muscles. To create your own 1-lb

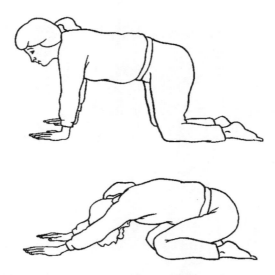

Figure 43: Slowly lean back on your feet and, with elbows straight, lower your head to the floor.

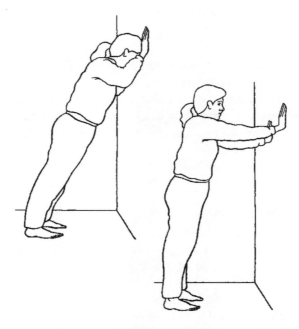

Figure 44: With feet away from the wall, bend your elbows and bring your forehead to the wall. Remember to keep your back straight.

weight, fill a small plastic detergent bottle with sand or pebbles. Or, you can hang a weighted bean bag (2 to 3 lb) over the broom handle or cane and use this to assist in strengthening.

Because the chest muscles are often weakened, especially if you have had a mastectomy, you can strengthen these muscles by doing push-ups while standing against a wall (Figure 44) or from a hands-and-knees position (Figure 45). First, stand with your feet about 2 feet (1/2 metre) apart. Place your hands on the wall, slightly outstretched, at the level of your head. Lean forward to touch your forehead against the wall. Push away slowly until your arms are fully extended. Repeat 8 to 12 times. To make the exercise harder, move your feet back further away from the wall.

The second type of push-up is from a hands-and-knees position (Figure 45). With your knees slightly apart and your hands placed slightly wider than your shoulders, lower your head until your nose touches the floor. Then, straighten your elbows until your arms are fully extended. Repeat 8 to 12 times.

If you have undergone axillary dissection

Because your lymphatic system has been interrupted as a result of the axillary dissection, it is advisable to wear a compression sleeve on your affected arm when doing weight-training involving more than 10 to 15 pounds (or any other strenuous upper body exercises). This is especially true if using weight-lifting equipment. When using weight machines such as a bench press or latissimus pull-down, start with the smallest weight possible (10 pounds) and increase very gradually. The greatest benefit is derived from weight-training if it is done at least twice a week with a minimum of 8 to 12 repetitions of each exercise.

Aerobic or conditioning exercises for cardiovascular fitness

Overall heart and lung fitness is important to promote health at any age or at any time in your life. Regular aerobic exercise can promote a good night's sleep, improve your overall sense of well-being, assist you in maintaining your ideal body weight, and keep your heart and lungs working effectively.

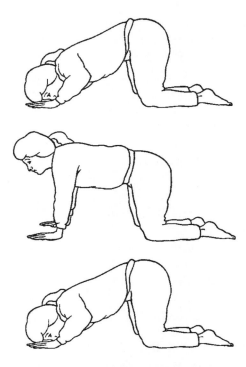

Figure 45: With knees slightly apart and hands wider than your shoulders, do a push-up, lowering your head until it touches the floor.

In order to gain maximum benefit, you should exercise continuously for 20 to 60 minutes per session, at least three to five days a week. Activities that involve large muscle groups, such as brisk walking, jogging, swimming, cycling, rowing, or skating, have the greatest benefit.

If you have not done regular exercise before, start out slowly and gradually. Walk four times around a quarter-mile track at your local high school and time yourself. If you don't like walking on a track, use your car to measure the distance of a pleasant walk through your neighbourhood. Or, walking on a treadmill in a community center allows you to time your walking speed and measure the distance walked. Continue to walk one mile, three to five times a week, but try to gradually increase your walking speed. When you can walk a mile in 15 or 16 minutes, increase your distance to one and a half miles.

Because women who have had breast cancer are usually advised not to take hormone replacement therapy, they will not have the protective benefits that estrogen replacement provides for the heart and bones. Therefore, both aerobic exercise (to improve heart function) and strengthening exercises (to increase bone density) are particularly important. Either a physical therapist or an exercise specialist can suggest a conditioning program for you to enhance your heart and bone health.

Scar tissue massage

It is important to loosen or 'break up' the scar tissue caused by breast cancer surgery, both to promote healing and minimize adhesions to the tissues underneath. Once your surgical wounds have healed and are no longer painful (usually four to six weeks after surgery), you can begin gently massaging the scar line using small, circular motions with the pads of your fingers. As the scars become less tender, use deeper pressure to try to loosen up the scar tissue.

You can use aloe vera lotion or another favorite body lotion for the massage. Some women like to do the massage while bathing or just after a bath. A physical therapist or a massage therapist can show you how to do the deep friction massage along the scar line. Ideally, scar tissue massage should be continued daily for at least one to two years after surgery.

Lymphedema

Women who have had axillary dissection can develop lymphedema (swelling) in the affected arm. Lymphedema occurs because the lymph fluid, which bathes the tissues in your arm to keep them free of infections, can no longer leave the arm through its normal channels in your armpit which can become disrupted during treatment. About 7% to 12% of women who have had axillary dissection will develop permanent lymphedema, usually within four months after their treatment. Some women (7%) develop transient (or temporary) lymphedema which disappears within a few months after breast cancer treatment.

It is therefore important that you report any sensations of puffiness or heaviness in your arm to your physical therapist or doctor. Ideally, you should have the circumference of both your arms measured before your breast cancer treatment and on a regular basis afterward. Either a physical therapist or your doctor can take the measurements using a tape measure at four specific points on your arm: at the knuckles, wrist, and 10 cm below and 15 cm above the elbow. Any single measurement that increases by more than 2 cm should be carefully monitored, with treatment begun for lymphedema.

Treating lymphedema

If you develop lymphedema you will need help from physicians, physical therapists, nurses, massage therapists and, sometimes, psychosocial counselors if the condition of your arm is causing you to be depressed.

For temporary lymphedema, elevation of the arm, a compression sleeve worn with activity, light massage given by a physical therapist or massage therapist, and close monitoring may be all that is required. Permanent lymphedema, however, requires constant care. Compression therapy, which involves the use of a compression garment and pump, works well. Compression pump therapy can be carried out several times a week or as needed. Physical therapists specializing in lymphedema care offer pump therapy and compression garments, as do many cancer centers. Also, a compression sleeve, with or without a gauntlet for hand swelling, needs to be worn during waking hours or while doing exercises.

A form of massage to stimulate lymphatic drainage, called manual lymph drainage (MLD) or manual lymph treatment (MLT), is gaining in popularity. It often involves bandaging and special exercises and is usually carried out by massage therapists. Complex physical therapy (CPT) or complex decongestive therapy (CDP) is a four-week treatment program which combines MLD, bandaging, exercises, support garments, and skin care counseling to control lymphedema.

Lymphedema is easier to control if you are not overweight and if you exercise regularly. It used to be said that, if you have lymphedema you shouldn't do active exercise with your arm, such as playing tennis, squash, lifting weights, rowing, or cross-country skiing. However, exercise and lymphedema have been poorly studied. Your arm will certainly tell you what activities it doesn't like, but it is highly recommended that you wear a compression sleeve with vigorous upper body exercise.

Avoid scratches, burns, cuts and bruises to your involved arm. When you need procedures to be done, such as having blood drawn, intravenous lines started or injections given, have them done on your healthy arm. Also, injuries can cause swelling or infection which is not handled well by the stagnant lymphatic system in your affected arm. Therefore, always be on the lookout for signs of infection in your arm (painful redness to your skin) and get immediate treatment. The infections are almost always caused by streptococcal bacteria and respond well to penicillin. You should always have some antibiotics on hand to be taken at the first sign of infections, especially if you are traveling to a remote area.

Preventing lymphedema

The following are key points for helping to prevent lymphedema, especially if you have had axillary dissection.

- Try to maintain an ideal body weight because obesity is a risk factor for lymphedema.
- Avoid having your blood pressure taken, blood drawn, injections or vaccinations, or intravenous lines started in the involved arm.
- Keep the skin of your arm clean and avoid injury, cuts, burns or infection.
- Consider wearing a compression sleeve when lifting heavy weights or engaging in vigorous upper body exercise, such as cross-country skiing, rowing or tennis. It used to be thought that you shouldn't do active exercise, but that advice has changed in recent years.
- Report any signs of arm swelling to your health-care provider immediately.

CHAPTER THIRTY-FIVE

Reconstructive surgery

by Patricia Clugston, MD,
and Richard Warren, MD

Should I or shouldn't I?

MANY WOMEN OPT FOR breast reconstruction, but many still choose not to have it done. In the latter case, they are simply relieved to be rid of their cancer and cannot imagine going through any further surgery. For other women, however, wearing an external prosthesis (see page 133) can be unsatisfactory, impractical and often bothersome. Reconstruction is an attractive option for women who feel this way. The most common reason for breast reconstruction is the psychological desire to feel 'whole' again. The goal of reconstructive surgery is to restore self-image and self-confidence and improve quality of life.

Breast reconstruction is an option for most women facing mastectomy. Occasionally, a patient's poor health or poor prognosis from their disease means that they cannot be considered for this operation. Also, some women are emotionally unprepared to undergo further surgery, with its related risks and potential complications. Women seeking breast reconstruction need to be physically and mentally healthy, must understand the associated risks and complications, and be motivated from within. They should not be undertaking reconstruction to please others in their lives.

Breast cancer treatment always takes precedence

The first goal of breast reconstruction is not to interfere with the treatment of the patient's breast cancer. A plastic surgeon may be consulted before the breast cancer surgery, and may do the reconstruction at the time of the mastectomy. The breast cancer surgeon, plastic surgeon and oncologist should ensure that the cancer treatment program is not adversely affected by the planned reconstruction. Also, reconstruction that is done following the cancer surgery should not interfere with detection of possible recurrence of the cancer on the chest or elsewhere in the body.

The first visit to the plastic surgeon

The initial referral to a plastic surgeon is usually arranged by the patient's breast surgeon, family physician or her oncologist. The patient will be asked questions about her expectations, desires, and general health, and a brief physical examination will be done. The available reconstructive options will be discussed and the preferred option for the individual patient will be explained in greater detail. The patient should ask questions to understand the options available, details of the proposed surgical procedure, the degree of pain involved, the recovery time, and the risks. She should expect the surgeon to provide diagrams and photographs or introductions to other patients so that she can have a realistic sense of the possible results and what to expect during the postoperative recovery period. Breast reconstruction is an inexact science, and while every surgeon has produced excellent results, possible postoperative complications and patient factors may contribute to a result that falls somewhat short.

Factors that affect the choice of reconstructive procedure

Reconstruction is designed to correct defects left by surgery. The type of procedure recommended will depend largely on the extent of the breast cancer surgery (see Chapter 19), but other factors also influence the choice of procedure and the expected cosmetic result. These will differ from one woman to another and include the amount and looseness of the skin, direction and length of the original surgical scar, the amount of fat under the skin, the possibility of skin changes caused by radiotherapy, and the shape and size of the other breast. Another factor that can also influence the overall reconstructive options is whether the procedure is done at the time of mastectomy (immediate reconstruction) or at some time following recovery (delayed reconstruction).

Surgical techniques

There are a variety of reconstructive techniques. No single technique is right for everyone. The choice of method will depend on the combination of the woman's wishes, the surgeon's preference, the type and extent of deformity, and the nature of the opposite breast. The various possibilities are outlined below in order of increasing complexity.

Implants

The simplest method of reconstruction is the insertion of a breast implant at the site of the original breast. This can be done either at the time of the mastectomy or any time later. This technique is most appropriate for patients who have enough of their own tissue remaining to cover the implant adequately, and for whom the implant alone will match the appearance of the other breast. This form of reconstruction is suitable when the opposite breast to be matched is relatively small and non-sagging, and the difference in the amount of skin between the two sides is minimal. Breast implants can be inserted in patients who have undergone a partial, a simple, or a modified radical mastectomy.

The implant is typically placed through a portion of the old incision, against the ribs, tucked underneath the pectoralis muscle. Because the muscle has to be present, this method is not appropriate for reconstruction after a radical mastectomy. The surgery is done under general anesthetic and usually involves a brief hospitalization. Postoperatively, there may be drains in place to remove any fluid build-up, and there will be more pain than from the original mastectomy. Possible problems include an infection, bleeding or problems related to the implant itself, which are discussed further on in this chapter. The most common disadvantage with this form of reconstruction is failure to achieve a similar shape to the opposite breast, both at the time of surgery and as the natural breast ages.

Tissue expander

A tissue expander is a device that looks like an empty plastic bag with an attached or incorporated valve. As with the implant, it is placed behind the pectoralis muscle. In the weeks following surgery, the expander is inflated using a small amount of saline (salt water). The idea is that after the surgical site has healed, the bag can be enlarged gradually by injecting salt water into the valve once or twice a week. Like the abdominal skin during pregnancy, the skin of the chest will stretch as the 'pseudo-breast' enlarges. Usually, this process goes on for one or two months in order to overstretch the skin to a size larger than the normal breast. Then, a second operation is done to remove the expander and replace it with a permanent breast implant (Figure 46).

This technique is appropriate for women who don't have enough skin remaining to allow insertion of an implant large enough to match the volume or shape of the other breast. Many surgeons who use this technique believe that by overstretching the skin, there will be a more natural droop to the breast after placement of the permanent implant.

Complications of this technique are the same as for the simple insertion of an implant. The one clear disadvantage of this method is that it involves two operations (as do most breast reconstructions) and extra visits to a doctor's office for the fluid injections.

The problem of capsular contracture

By far the most common problem with breast implants and tissue expanders is the phenomenon of 'capsular contracture' in which a layer of scar tissue forms around the implant and squeezes it into a firm ball. This was a much more common problem when silicone gel implants were the preferred implant for breast reconstruction. The chance of developing capsular

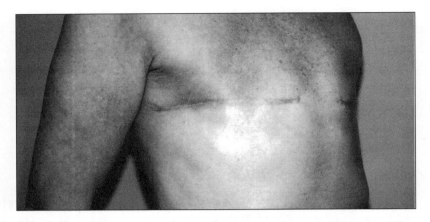

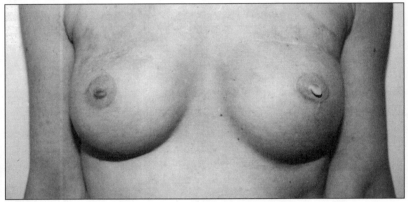

Figure 46: The result of breast and nipple reconstruction of both breasts. Tissue expanders were used to stretch the skin from the preoperative stage (upper) until there was sufficient room for the implants to be inserted. At a later operation the nipples were reconstructed (lower).

contracture is higher (about 50%) if the patient has previously had radiation to the mastectomy site. With saline implants in the absence of previous radiation, the incidence of contracture is approximately 10% to 20%. Some patients may require further surgery to correct it.

Other problems include bleeding, infection, nerve damage and, with saline implants, the potential of a leak leading to deflation and the necessity of replacing the implant with a new one.

Over the past decade, textured saline implants and tissue expanders were introduced in the hope of decreasing the risk of capsular contracture and optimizing the shape of the reconstructed breast. However, there is a tendency for these devices to become relatively immobile on the chest wall and patient satisfaction has been low except in patients in whom reconstruction of both breasts is required.

Myocutaneous flaps

A third type of reconstruction involves the use of 'myocutaneous flaps.' This requires the movement of a piece of tissue that includes skin, fat and muscle from one part of the body to another. The rationale for the use of myocutaneous flaps is that by using the body's own tissue, a more natural-feeling breast may be created, avoiding the complications related to implants. However, there is a trade-off, since the more complex surgery involves increased risks, scarring, potential donor site problems and increased recovery time.

In one type of myocutaneous flap operation, the latissimus dorsi muscle (the large triangular muscle from the back) along with the overlying skin is moved into the mastectomy area. For some women, enough tissue can be transferred from the back to create a good breast size (medium B cup). If a larger breast is required, this procedure can be combined with a small implant to optimize volume. However, this operation leaves a scar and a contour deformity on the back and eliminates the latissimus as a functioning muscle in the back (Figure 47). Surprisingly, most patients are not aware of this lost function afterwards. The hospital stay is approximately three to four days. Often, the patient is discharged with a drain in the back donor site and will require home care until this is removed.

Currently, the most commonly used flap technique is the 'Transverse Rectus Abdominus Muscle' flap, know as the TRAM flap. Of all the options, this type of surgery will produce the best results for those patients who are highly motivated, have a suitable abdomen, and are willing to tolerate a longer recovery phase. This method uses a large section of skin and fat from the lower abdomen (belly) along with a portion of one of the rectus (sit-up) muscles which provides the blood supply to

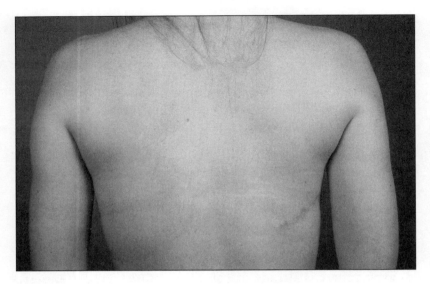

Figure 47: Surgical scar and muscle contour defect on the back of a woman who had a right-sided latissimus dorsi flap reconstruction.

the tissue. A breast mound is fashioned out of the skin and fat which has been brought up from the abdomen (Figure 48).

The abdominal defect where the muscle is taken is repaired with sutures, and sometimes requires reinforcement with surgical mesh. Postoperatively, the patient is mobilized slowly and typically spends four to six days in hospital. The abdominal area is more uncomfortable than the chest as a result of muscle spasms. Drains will be present at the breast site as well as in the abdomen, and will gradually be removed as the amount of drainage decreases. About 50% of patients leave hospital with one abdominal drain still in place, which is removed by the home-care nurse a few days after drainage has decreased. Recovery time is usually 6 to 12 weeks, depending on the patient. Strenuous abdominal activity is discouraged for 6 to 8 weeks. The amount of time off work averages 6 to 12 weeks; however, some patients require more time.

Although using the body's own tissues sounds attractive, this is a complex method of breast reconstruction, with additional possible complications, including abdominal wall hernia (about 2%), part of the flap not surviving (5% to 20% in non-

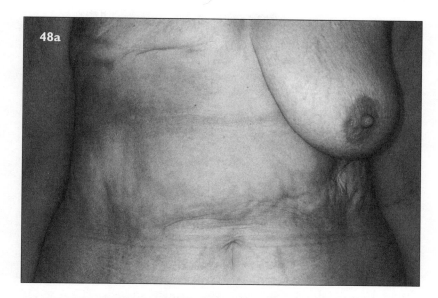

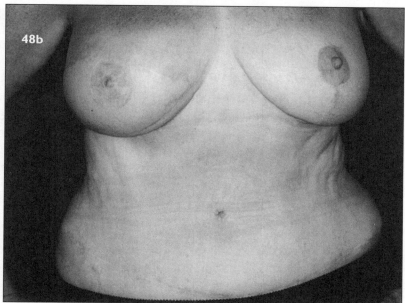

Figure 48: Preoperative (48a) and one year postoperative (48b) appearance of a woman with a delayed TRAM flap reconstruction and left reduction mammoplasty carried out for symmetry. The abdominal scar is just visible above the panty line. At a second operation the right-sided nipple was created.

smokers, higher in smokers), thrombophlebitis (formation of blood clots in the veins), healing problems in the abdominal site and postoperative lung problems (rare). If reconstruction is done at the time of mastectomy, there is an increased risk of a portion of the mastectomy flap not surviving in about 10% to 15% of patients. Although this may not ultimately affect the overall reconstructive result, it requires extra wound care and dressings to the area over a period of several weeks.

Women at highest risk for complications are those with large, heavy breasts, diabetics, smokers, those with chronic lung disease, immune arthritic conditions, or those who have had previous radiation therapy to the breast or chest wall. These patients should only be considered candidates for flap surgery if the surgeon has extensive experience in these techniques and the patient is extremely motivated and understanding of the potential risks. Most surgeons require patients to quit smoking beforehand, ideally two to three months prior to TRAM flap surgery. Another issue which may prevent the use of this method is the presence of other surgical scars in the abdomen which may have disrupted the necessary blood supply to the abdominal tissue.

A side benefit of TRAM flap breast reconstruction is a free 'tummy tuck' (Figure 48). However, if a patient has had a previous tummy tuck procedure, they can no longer be considered for this surgery. Previous abdominal liposuction can also increase the risks associated with the TRAM flap procedure, and may have reduced the available fatty tissue to an inadequate volume for this type of operation.

Second stage breast reconstruction

Most breast reconstruction should be viewed as a two-staged surgical procedure. The first step is to create a new breast mound using one of the techniques already discussed. The second procedure is planned four to six months later and should be viewed as a minor procedure to optimize symmetry between the two breasts and reconstruct a nipple. If the original reconstruction was a flap procedure, then minor scar revisions are usually done at this time.

Nipple reconstruction

Most women who seek breast reconstruction are happy once a breast mound has been created but, if offered, will opt to have completion of their reconstruction by the creation of a nipple and areola. There are various techniques available to achieve this, and to a large extent the technique selected will depend on the preference and experience of the plastic surgeon. Typically, the projecting nipple can be made from small flaps of tissue raised up locally off the previously created breast mound (Figure 48), or it can be taken from the opposite nipple as a graft if the opposite nipple is large. The more darkly pigmented areola can be fashioned from a portion of the opposite areola or a skin graft from high on the inside of the thigh, or it can simply be tattooed.

Nipple-areola reconstruction is relatively minor surgery. The main problems relate to partial graft failure, loss of projection of the reconstructed nipple and mismatched color.

Matching the breast exactly

Paradoxically, the easiest situation for achieving identical-looking breasts (symmetry) with mastectomy reconstruction is when both breasts are reconstructed (Figure 46). Although the goal of reconstructing one breast is to match the normal breast, an exact match is seldom possible. To get a close match, the normal breast may need to be altered. This may require uplift (mastopexy) or reduction of the normal breast. Both of these procedures create some scars on the normal breast, and introduce some risks and potential complications. Despite this, symmetry surgery of the opposite breast is generally very well tolerated and often gives the patient a more youthful, less heavy and droopy breast that more closely matches the reconstructed breast (Figure 48).

Timing of breast reconstruction

Traditionally, breast reconstruction after mastectomy was delayed for a period of time, often a year, to allow time to complete additional therapies such as radiation and chemotherapy, and to allow the woman to recover mentally and physically

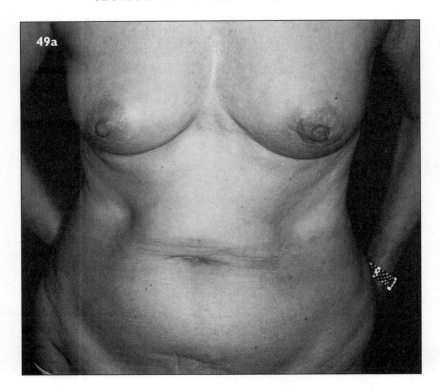

Figures 49a and b: Preoperative (49a) and one year postoperative (49b) comparison of a woman who had an immediate TRAM flap reconstruction of the left breast. A skin-sparing mastectomy was done through the small circular scar surrounding the left areola in 49b, and the patient's own nipple and

from her ordeal before she proceeded with more extensive surgery. This wait is no longer thought to be medically necessary and some patients now undergo immediate reconstruction. In these cases, the reconstruction procedure is done at the same time as the mastectomy. Advantages of this include reducing the number of operations and reducing the necessary recovery time and time off work, avoiding the body image disturbance and grief reaction that many patients suffer after mastectomy, and optimizing the overall cosmetic result by allowing a skin-sparing (skin-saving) mastectomy (Figure 49). However, despite the improved cosmetic results that are often attainable with immediate reconstruction, patients in this group are often more criti-

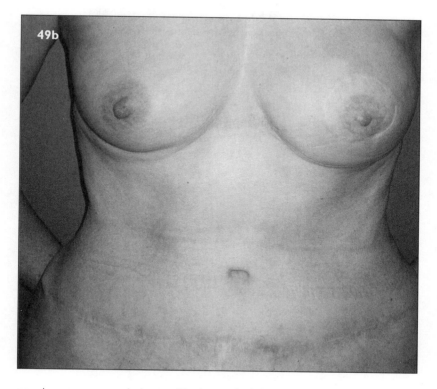

areola was removed along with the underlying breast tissue. The breast mound is composed of tissue transferred from the site of the new abdominal scar. In a second-stage operation, the nipple and areola in 49b were fashioned surgically and with tattooing.

cal of their reconstruction result compared with those who have had to live with a mastectomy deformity prior to reconstruction.

Disadvantages of immediate reconstruction include the coordination of two surgeons, a longer operation, and a potentially increased number of complications. Some oncologists prefer that if additional therapies such as chemotherapy and radiation are likely going to be given postoperatively and a patient is at high risk for wound healing complications (smokers, diabetics, obese patients, large-breasted patients), then these patients may be better suited for delayed reconstruction. Timing, then, is a decision that should be made in consultation with the patient, the oncologic surgeon and an oncologist involved in the patient's care.

Are breast implants dangerous?

Over the years a number of different materials have been tried for reconstructing breasts, including sponges, human fat, injected substances, and breast implants. Other than the use of the patient's own tissue, such as with the TRAM flap, only breast implants have been successful. However, their use has become controversial. Invented in the 1960s, breast implants have been manufactured in many forms, the basic design being a bag of silicone rubber filled with some sort of soft material. The most widely used type has been one filled with a silicone liquid or a gel, while another type is filled with salt water (saline). A third type of implant was the 'bi-lumen,' a hybrid type consisting of silicone gel surrounded by a second bag of saline.

In recent years it has become apparent that implants filled with silicone gel leak microscopic amounts of silicone over time, and there have been reports of health problems, mainly autoimmune diseases such as arthritis, possibly related to the silicone gel. At present, extensive studies are being done to determine the validity of these concerns, but the absolute risk of these complications appears to be very small. Nevertheless, health authorities in the United States and Canada have taken the safest position, deciding to remove silicone gel implants from the marketplace in 1991. In the United States, silicone gel-filled implants are still available under certain circumstances and on special request. There does not appear to be any need to remove a silicone gel prosthesis if it is not causing the woman any problems.

The standard implant used in North America today is the saline-filled breast implant. Saline implants are considered safe because a leak will only release salt water, which is the same as the major fluid component of our blood. This means that if the fluid leaks it is readily absorbed by the body without any health risk other than the need to replace the implant.

Life Style Issues

CHAPTER THIRTY-SIX

Nutrition

by Cheryl Kutynec, MSc, RDN,
and Shirley Hobenshield, RDN

WE EAT TO SATISFY a complex set of needs — emotional, cultural, sensual and, of course, nutritional. Eating well, in every sense of the word, is one of the most supportive things that a woman with breast cancer can do for herself.

What is a healthy diet?

Healthy eating means choosing a wide variety of foods that are low in fat and high in dietary fiber. In North America, this means focusing more on plant-based foods, including whole grain cereals and breads, vegetables, fruit and legumes (beans), and choosing smaller amounts of lean meat, chicken and fish as well as low-fat dairy products.

A healthy diet also means achieving balance, that is, eating foods in the right proportions to make sure that your needs for essential nutrients such as protein, vitamins and minerals are being met. The Healthy Eating Plan on page 245 provides a broad outline of the groups of foods that should be included in a balanced diet.

Is there a link between diet and breast cancer?

Among other factors, diet may influence the risk of developing breast cancer. Many scientists feel that a diet that is high in fat and limited in fruits and vegetables may increase this risk. In North America, research studies are ongoing to see whether women who follow a low-fat diet are less likely to develop breast cancer. In addition, a diet rich in soy foods (soy beans, tofu, soy milk) may be protective for the development of breast cancer.

Once you have had breast cancer, changing your diet at this time may also be beneficial. It is possible that eating a diet low in fat may reduce the risk of breast cancer recurrence. Research is beginning to evaluate the safety and potential role of soy foods for women with a history of breast cancer.

Is there a special diet to follow while undergoing breast cancer therapy?

You should follow a healthy diet, making sure that you are getting enough calories and protein each day. Your body also needs adequate amounts of a variety of nutrients to help healing after surgery or while going through radiation therapy or chemotherapy. You will get enough protein and calories by following the Healthy Eating Plan on page 245. If you find it difficult to eat a variety of vegetables, fruits and whole grain foods, then a daily multivitamin/mineral tablet is recommended.

If there are days when solid foods don't appeal to you, you may want to try the recipes for high-calorie, high-protein drinks listed below.

High-protein milk shake

250 mL	skim or 1% milk	1 cup
50 mL	skim milk powder	1/4 cup
1 scoop	light ice cream, ice milk or frozen yogurt	1/2 cup

Blend until smooth. Chill before serving. Makes one serving. This recipe may be varied by adding fruit such as 125 mL (1/2 cup) of berries or peaches, or 1/2 banana. Per serving: 1200 kJ (285 calories), 19 g protein, 4 g fat (using skim milk and ice milk).

Tofu fruit shake

300 g	soft tofu	1 package
175 mL	sweetened soy milk	3/4 cup
75 mL	frozen fruit juice concentrate	1/3 cup
45 mL	honey	3 tbsp
1	ripe banana	

Blend until smooth. Chill before serving. Makes two servings. This recipe may also be varied by adding fruit. Per serving: 1500 kJ (360 calories), 11 g protein, 6 g fat.

If you're having chemotherapy

During chemotherapy, nausea, a sore mouth, taste changes and mild diarrhea may occur.

Ease nausea with starchy snacks and light drinks

Nausea is best controlled by a combination of medications and certain foods. Dry, starchy foods like crackers and dry cereals, nibbled often, can help minimize that empty stomach feeling that can make nausea worse. Fluids like flat ginger ale, weak tea, diluted fruit juice or just plain ice water are generally better tolerated than milk shakes, coffee or very sweet juices. Keeping a thermos or giant cup close by can help remind you of the importance of drinking lots of fluid during chemotherapy.

If the smell of cooking food makes nausea worse, try to avoid being in the kitchen, if possible. If this is not realistic, it's a good idea to stock up on store-bought or homemade frozen meals that can be easily reheated.

Soothe mouth sores

If mouth sores occur during chemotherapy, certain foods should be avoided until the sores heal, such as oranges and grapefruit, salty or spicy foods, or rough foods, like toast. Many women find frozen yogurt, ice milk and blenderized shakes very soothing. (See recipes for shakes listed above.)

If foods taste different

Some women notice that certain foods taste different during chemotherapy. For example, meat may taste bitter or metallic.

If this happens, choose more mild-tasting, high-protein foods like eggs, milk or tofu to make eating more enjoyable. Food cravings may also occur. For instance, some women crave 'comfort' foods such as rice pudding during treatment. Many women report that fruits and certain vegetables are often the most appealing foods.

If you have diarrhea or gas

Mild diarrhea and gas can be a problem. You can minimize diarrhea by limiting your intake of alcohol, strong coffee, strong tea and cola, and by eating less high-fiber foods. Excess gas can be at least partially controlled by eating less gas-forming foods like legumes (beans) and vegetables from the cabbage family, such as cabbage, Brussels sprouts and broccoli.

If you're having radiation therapy

Most women undergoing radiation therapy for breast cancer report very little disturbance in their usual eating habits. However, fatigue can make food preparation more of a chore than usual. It's a good idea to have on hand a variety of convenience foods like frozen dinners. Meals can be simple but still nutritious — a sandwich or a bowl of cereal with milk and fruit is fine. Women whose radiation treatment involves the throat area can develop temporary soreness and a feeling of a lump or discomfort during swallowing. Eating soft, moist foods is helpful, such as poached eggs, creamed fish, chicken stew or fruit yogurt. An even smoother consistency can be achieved by putting foods through a blender. Very hot foods such as tea or soup can make a sore throat worse.

What about gaining weight during treatment?

Regardless of the type of treatment you are receiving, unwanted weight gain is quite common. It most often occurs in premenopausal women being treated with chemotherapy and/or hormone therapy. Weight gain may also be increased by naturally occurring or treatment-related menopause. The exact cause of unwanted weight gain is unclear, but it may be due to a number of factors, including decreased physical activity, eating frequently to control nausea, eating as an antidote to boredom or psychological distress, or because of an increased appetite or food cravings. If you have recently quit smoking, you may also notice that your weight has increased.

How can weight gain be managed?

It's not a good idea to try to lose weight during treatment because it puts unnecessary stress on the body and can actually slow down healing. A better goal is to maintain your weight until treatment is complete. You can do this by limiting high-fat foods and eating more fruits, vegetables and whole grains, which are low in calories. If frequent eating is necessary to control nausea, low-fat foods are a good choice, like crackers, cereal and skim milk, bread and jam, and canned soft fruits. If you have always had difficulty maintaining your weight, you may also consider other life-style changes, including being more physically active to achieve a healthy body weight. Women who are taking the drug treatment megestrol acetate (Megace®) may find weight control especially difficult, but a healthy, low-fat, high-fiber diet can help. Ask your doctor or nutritionist for more advice.

Are extra vitamins and minerals helpful during treatment?

It's not yet clear whether the use of large doses of vitamins and minerals help in cancer treatment. Those who support their use point out that since cancer treatments can depress the immune system, taking vitamins and minerals could help restore immune function. Although a number of nutrients are required for the immune system to function properly (including vitamins A, C, E, B_6, beta-carotene, folic acid, zinc and iron), too much of a good thing is not necessarily better and can be harmful. For example, too much zinc actually depresses the immune system.

Another theory is that the antioxidant vitamins (vitamins C, E, and beta-carotene) are required to help repair cells damaged during cancer treatment. This is being studied, but there's not enough evidence as yet to indicate that supplements of antioxidant vitamins do help in cancer treatment. However, dark green and orange vegetables and a variety of fruits are a good source of the antioxidant vitamins C and beta-carotene, and are recommended as part of a healthy diet. Eating large amounts of these fruits and vegetables is not harmful. The only side effect to note is a harmless yellow coloring to the skin (but not the eyes) that occurs when people eat a large amount of carrots or other orange vegetables.

If you are interested in using high doses of vitamin or mineral supplements, it is a good idea to discuss this with your physicians and nutritionist to confirm that these supplements can be used safely along with other treatments you may be receiving.

Once treatment's over, keep eating well

Even after treatment is over, it makes sense to continue eating less fat and more fruits, vegetables and whole grain foods. If you haven't already made these changes to your diet, this is the best time to start. Besides having a possible link to breast cancer risk, too much fat in the diet has been linked to heart disease and obesity. By simply becoming aware of where fat is found in your diet, you can take steps to reduce your fat intake. Try to remove visible fats on chicken or meat wherever you can. Also, limit the amount of fat you add to foods by skipping butter of margarine on sandwiches, using light salad dressings, and using extra herbs and spices instead of cream sauces.

Finally, be aware of hidden fat. This is the trickiest: it's found in foods like cookies, cakes, chips, ice cream and cheese. You can limit hidden fat by reading food labels carefully and choosing alternatives such as low-fat cheese. Ask your nutritionist for further advice.

For more advice on nutrition

You can obtain further advice about nutrition by contacting a registered dietitian at your regional cancer center or community hospital. As well, in some places there are nutrition hotlines staffed by qualified dietitians. Check with your local dietetic association about resources in your area.

In the United States, the phone number of the Consumer Nutrition Hotline of the American Dietetic Association is 1-800-366-1655. Dial-a-Dietitian in British Columbia can be reached at 1-800-667-DIET.

The Additional Reading section lists several cookbooks devoted to lower-fat, higher-fiber meals. The recipes are easy to follow and most importantly, taste great!

Healthy eating plan

In one day you should eat:

5 to 12 servings of grain products
5 to 10 servings of vegetables and fruit
2 to 4 servings of milk product
2 to 3 servings of meat and alternatives

Grain products (each is 1 serving)
- 1 slice of bread
- 1/2 a bagel or pita bread
- 1/2 cup (125 mL) of cooked pasta or rice
- 3/4 cup (175 mL) of cooked cereal
- 30 g of dry cereal (1/3 to 1 cup, depending on the type of cereal)

Vegetables and fruit (each is 1 serving)
- 1 medium-sized vegetable or fruit, such as one carrot, potato, apple, orange or banana
- 1/2 cup (125 mL) of vegetables or fruit, such as corn, broccoli, berries, peas, or applesauce
- 1 cup (250 mL) of salad
- 1/2 cup (125 mL) of juice

Milk products (each is 1 serving)
- 1 cup (250 mL) of milk
- 3/4 cup (175 g) of yogurt
- 2 ounces (50 g) of cheese
- 1 cup (250 mL) fortified soy beverage*

Meat and alternatives (each is 1 serving)
- 2-3 ounces (50-100 g)
- 1/3-2/3 can (50-100 g) of tuna or salmon
- 1/2-1 cup (125-250 mL) cooked legumes, e.g. beans, lentils, split peas
- 1/3 cup (100 g) tofu
- 1-2 eggs
- 2 tablespoons (30 mL) of nut or seed butter
- 3-4 tablespoons (45-60 mL) nuts or seeds

*Fortified soy beverage contains added calcium, vitamins A and D, riboflavin and B$_{12}$ and is available in some areas.

CHAPTER THIRTY-SEVEN

Stress and relaxation

by Lis Smith, CCH

What is stress?

STRESS IS WOVEN into the fabric of life. At healthy levels it challenges us and promotes activity, but when you feel 'overloaded' or 'lose control' then the stress level is no longer healthy. The uncertainty and fears surrounding a diagnosis of breast cancer can lead to a feeling of overload just when there is a great need to be 'in control' and it can threaten your well-being.

How much stress am I feeling?

Stress is a subjective response and is not expressed the same way in each person. When stress becomes too great the mind may say that you are 'coping,' but the body gives more accurate signals. If you recognize and acknowledge your own stress response you can begin to deal with it.

To assess your own response to stress, learn to scan your body while asking yourself questions. Start at the top of your head, searching for tightness between the brow and eyes. Are your lips pursed? Is your jaw clenched? Are your shoulders hunched up near your ears? Normally, one doesn't notice doing these things until alerted by a pounding headache or lower back pain at the end of the day caused by holding muscles so tense.

Do you feel a tightness in the throat, a constriction in the chest or a churning stomach? Are you breathing shallowly, using only the upper part of your chest? Does your heart beat fast? Some people notice that their sleep pattern is disturbed, and others eat more than they need because eating is comforting.

When in distress the mind doesn't focus and function the way it usually does. You may forget your own telephone number or an important appointment. Your thoughts may be dark and repetitive, and after only an hour's sleep you may lie awake for hours doing what has been so aptly called 'awfulizing.' Emotionally, you are not as steady as usual, and find yourself in tears over something that you would normally take in stride.

To be told to 'relax' at a time like this may seem unreasonable. You do know, however, that when you are not feeling the effects of an overload of stress, you find yourself filled with a tranquil energy and a sense of control. How do you achieve this elusive feeling, especially after a recent diagnosis of breast cancer?

How can I reduce stress and regain a sense of control?

Reading this book, gaining knowledge about breast cancer, is one practical way to help yourself find that sense of control. Also, finding someone simply to listen is of enormous value.

Research has shown that even twenty minutes a day of relaxation can have a beneficial effect on the body. It doesn't matter whether it is transcendental meditation or simply sitting quietly watching the birds at a feeder outside the window. Twenty minutes of steady walking or other exercise works for some people. Tai-Chi and yoga also use movement to bring the body and mind into a state of harmony. Meditation, in which the mind focuses on a particular word (mantra) or object (mandala), or simply focusing on the rising and falling of the breath stills the chattering mind and restores a sense of equilibrium. Anything that allows the body to be at ease and the mind to quieten a little appears to bring back balance and harmony. Think of the ocean. Even when a storm is raging, deep below there is a place where the water is calm. So it is with your own self. You need to find the way down to that place deep within yourself where you are calm and in control, even in the midst of chaos.

Women are used to being responsible for others and putting their own needs last. Giving yourself permission to take some time for yourself can be an important part of the healing process. Be your own good care-giver; it is okay to say 'yes' to your own needs.

The relaxation response

Relaxation is about tranquil energy and gaining a sense of control so that you can respond to situations and make good choices rather than just react. It is interesting that the ancient Chinese symbol for crisis has two components, one meaning 'danger,' the other meaning 'opportunity.' Gaining a sense of control gives you an opportunity to make creative choices.

The breath is the pulse of the mind. You can slow your racing thoughts simply by changing your breathing, especially by breathing from the bottom of the diaphragm instead of the shallow, tight breathing from high in the chest that usually accompanies stress. For example: take a comfortable, deep breath, hold it to the count of four and then let it out with a sigh. Repeat this four times. Feel how your shoulders release and your facial muscles soften. When you find yourself experiencing tension, remind yourself to take a sighing breath.

'Autogenics' is another way to occupy the thinking mind by getting it busy with repeated words such as 'My right arm is heavy, my right arm is warm.' By this repetition the mind starts to convince the body that its different parts are at ease. This feeling of bodily comfort induces a sense of calm control.

Another way to achieve the relaxation response is to imagine yourself in a beautiful place, perhaps in nature or a delightful room, or to relive the memory of a time of achievement and strength. This is the opposite of 'awfulizing,' as you use your body-mind connection to create sensations of peace and 'connectedness.' Audiotapes can also be very helpful by coaching you through these experiences (see Additional Reading).

'Quick fixes'

Sometimes finding even twenty minutes a day for relaxing seems like a tall order. You may wish to experiment with some 'quick fixes' which will help you become familiar with the healing benefits of relaxation.

Whenever you are particularly stressed you quite naturally do one of these 'quick fixes' already: you sigh. You can cultivate sighing as a way towards relaxation. After three or four comfortable sighing breaths you will find that the muscles of the face are more at ease, the chest feels more open and the shoulders are softer. Because one needs regular reminders to sigh, try putting little colored dots in all sorts of places such as on your steering wheel, on the telephone or on your purse. These dots can serve as triggers, reminders to take a breath, hold it to the count of four and then sigh the breath out. Do this throughout the day.

Another 'quick fix' is to practice a quick progressive muscle relaxation every time you sit down. Let tension flow from the top of your head out through the soles of your feet. Or take a 30-second vacation and recall a beautiful place or happy, carefree time.

Certain fragrances are known to soothe and elevate one's mood. Try a few drops of neroli oil, lavender, geranium or another fragrance which pleases you as you relax in a warm bath. Many health food stores and pharmacies carry aroma therapy products.

Increasingly, you will recognize the importance of your own role in the healing process, in partnership with your physicians and the treatments and medications offered. Learning your role can add a rich dimension to the power of the partnership.

What if Cancer Recurs?

CHAPTER THIRTY-EIGHT

Follow-up: Support, side effects and concerns about recurrence

OFTEN, IT IS ONLY at the end of treatment that women start to worry about the possibility of a relapse. 'What if the breast cancer recurs? When will it recur? What can I do to prevent it from coming back? What is my prognosis if it does relapse? Will I die? How long have I got?'

What are the goals of follow-up?

The aims of regular follow-up after treatment for breast cancer are to provide support, to assess, explain and manage any side effects from treatment, and to offer early detection of potentially curable new disease. These visits are also an opportunity to ask questions and discuss any new information that you are wondering about. Unfortunately, although there are many useful treatments that can be used if breast cancer recurs and is causing symptoms, there is no curative treatment if breast cancer is found in other organs, beyond the breast and lymph node regions. In follow-up, therefore, the doctors should be carefully looking for new disease in the breast or lymph nodes, including doing regular mammograms, but there is no value in doing a lot of other tests like chest x-rays, bone scans or blood tests.

What are the chances of a recurrence?

Recurrences occur because cells were left behind in the breast, lymph nodes or chest wall (a local recurrence) or cells got into the blood vessels and travelled to other parts of the body such as bones, liver or lungs (a systemic recurrence). The word for the movement of cancer cells is 'metastasize' and the new growths in other organs are called 'metastases.'

The risk of relapse is related to several factors, including whether the cancer is in situ or invasive, the size of the tumor, the clinical stage, and the presence and number of cancer-involved lymph nodes. Patients with in situ disease have a very low risk of the cancer recurring elsewhere in the body, but there is a possibility of local recurrence or of a cancer developing in the other breast.

For invasive cancers, the risk of relapse is related to the clinical stage (Chapter 17). In clinical stage I disease (a small tumor and no cancer found in the axillary lymph nodes), 75% to 95% of patients will be alive with no recurrence 10 years or longer after treatment. In more advanced stages the risk of relapse is greater. Approximately 50% of stage II patients and 75% of those with a locally advanced cancer will develop a recurrence either locally or elsewhere in the body in the first 10 years after treatment.

New therapies are being studied all over the world. Information is shared internationally so that women can gain access to new therapies quickly, hopefully improving these statistics so that over the next few years fewer women will suffer a relapse.

When should I worry about a new problem?

Most systemic recurrences cause symptoms; they are rarely silent. The symptoms depend on which organ is affected. For example, breast cancer that has travelled to the bones will often cause pain, while recurrences in the lungs may cause cough or shortness of breath. It is often difficult for a patient who has recently been diagnosed to know which symptoms might be indicative of recurrent disease and which symptoms are simply normal aches and pains. It takes time for a woman to start trusting her body again after a diagnosis of breast cancer. The worry about systemic relapse makes it hard to be at ease.

In general, symptoms of recurrence are more persistent than normal aches and pains and become progressively more severe. For example, a backache that's brought on by moving furniture usually feels bad for a day or two and then gradually gets better. Metastatic bone disease in the back may come on gradually, may come and go with activity and may respond to pain killers, but it will not go away completely and stay away. Instead, it will become more persistent. It is very common for women to be more aware of their bodies after a diagnosis of cancer. It is normal to think that an ache, for example in the leg, is due to cancer. However, if a pain comes and goes in 24 hours it is not likely to be cancer and you don't need to worry.

On the other hand, if you are worried about a new symptom, especially if it is persistent or getting worse, you should see your doctor. She will do an examination and order any investigations that may be necessary. If everything is normal and the symptoms continue to bother you, they may be due to something other than the breast cancer. Not all new symptoms mean a recurrence of breast cancer, but your doctor should evaluate them and arrive at a diagnosis.

How and by whom should I be followed?

All women, after a diagnosis of breast cancer, should have follow-up visits to provide information and support and to check for a local recurrence or metastasis. However, medical opinion differs on the best follow-up schedule, and women's needs also vary. Many women are more comfortable with frequent follow-up and the reassurance that there is no detectable recurrence. Other women find the follow-up visits cause unnecessary anxiety. It is important that the woman and her doctor agree on a schedule of follow-up which provides reassurance and support and detects most recurrences promptly, but allows the woman to return to normal living without feeling like an invalid.

It is not essential that you be followed at a cancer center. Many women receive excellent support and surveillance from their family physicians. It is important that you feel confident in the doctor's ability to listen to you and examine you, particularly the treated breast if you had breast-conserving surgery. If you are seeing several different physicians, space out the visits to avoid duplication. For example, if you are seeing two doctors, see each one annually but one in the spring and one in the fall so that you are examined every six months rather than twice in the fall. Be sure your doctors have an effective means of communicating with each other about the results of their examinations and their recommendations about your care.

Unfortunately, we must acknowledge that with treatments available today there is very little advantage to the early detection of a systemic recurrence, and performing lots of x-rays and blood tests to look for metastases is not recommended. The situation is different for local recurrence which may be curable with further surgery. Also, it is useful to detect the development of a second breast cancer in the opposite breast as early as possible since this too may be curable. Therefore, regular mammograms are the only 'routine' test recommended for women who feel well after treatment for breast cancer.

How often should I have follow-up visits and what should happen?

We recommend a first follow-up visit about six weeks after the treatment (surgery, chemotherapy and radiation therapy) is complete. Then, you should have visits approximately every six months. At each visit, the physician should ask about side effects, including your level of appetite, energy, menopausal symptoms, pain, arm swelling and your emotional health. If you are taking tamoxifen, the physician should inquire if you have had any vaginal spotting or bleeding. You should expect to be examined, at least in the region of the breasts, arms, neck, chest and abdomen. This visit will also be an opportunity for you to ask questions. You should mention any new symptoms or change in how your body is functioning such as bony aches and pains, cough or shortness of breath, nausea and weight loss, or new lumps and bumps, since these may be indications of recurrent disease.

Blood tests are often normal despite evidence of a local or even systemic recurrence and are not recommended as part of the regular checkups unless a woman has noticed a new symptom or change in her body. Routine bone or liver scans are not recommended in women without symptoms. Chest x-rays should be done if there are any symptoms that relate to the lungs but not as part of regular follow-up.

Mammograms

We recommend that a set of baseline mammograms be done approximately six months after the completion of treatment. It is highly unlikely that any cancer recurrence will be detected this soon, but most of the breast changes due to surgery and/or radiation should have settled. This 6-month study will serve as a 'baseline' of the new 'normal' appearance of the breast and will be used for comparison with future mammograms. Subsequently, mammograms should be done annually. Not all mammogram abnormalities are cancer. After radiation and surgery there may be changes in the breast such as scarring or swelling which can be monitored with regular mammograms. Mammograms of the unaffected breast should also be performed once a year.

For how long should I have regular follow-up visits?

Most recurrences of breast cancer occur in the first two to five years after treatment, but they can occur even 10 to 20 years later. Although five years is not a 'magical' cure date, we recommend regular visits to a doctor every six months until five years after treatment and then annually as long as you are well. If cancer recurs, the schedule of visits to your doctor will be individualized depending on the kinds of problems the cancer may be causing, the types and response to treatments you are receiving, and your preferences.

Your responsibilities

You are responsible for some aspects of the follow-up. You may want to learn how to do a thorough monthly breast self-examination. This includes examining the uninvolved breast and the radiated breast or the chest wall if a mastectomy has been done. Any new findings or changes should be reported to your doctor. It's important to know that not all changes are due to cancer recurrence. Many women develop thickened areas or redness in a radiated breast, or thickened areas along the scar. Often, it is difficult to know if the thickening is cancerous or not, and a mammogram or biopsy may be necessary. You should show your doctor the area of concern and he or she will do a physical examination and order additional tests if necessary. You should report any new symptoms or problems to your doctor, and remind any new physicians that you see of your history of breast cancer.

CHAPTER THIRTY-NINE

Treatment of
a local recurrence

WHEN THE CANCER RECURS at or near the site of the original breast cancer many patients are surprised and confused. How can the cancer recur after surgery, radiation and chemotherapy? There are a number of theories, including: 1) that cancer cells are left in the skin after surgery, 2) that cancer cells remain in the muscles or lymphatic system of the chest wall after surgery in an area that was not removed with a mastectomy or partial mastectomy, and 3) that the cancer cells were present in the blood stream before the operation and returned to the chest wall after the surgery. Each of these theories may be important in an individual case.

What are the signs of local or regional recurrences?

A local or regional recurrence refers to a relapse of breast cancer in the area that includes the breast, the armpit, the skin or chest wall after mastectomy and the surrounding lymph nodes. Radiation to the breast, chest wall and lymph node regions can significantly reduce the occurrence of relapse in these areas. Possible signs of local or regional relapse include new lumps, 'thickening' or rashes in the breast, chest wall, armpit or above the collarbone. Recurrence in the lymph nodes in the armpit or behind the collarbone may cause shoulder pain, arm swelling, pain that shoots down the arm, or numbness and weakness in the hand or arm due to cancer pinching the nerves that extend down into the hand and arm from the neck. Any of these symptoms should prompt a physician evaluation.

How are local recurrences treated?

Local relapses often require local treatments such as surgery or radiation, especially if no other recurrence is detected elsewhere in the body. However, if there is evidence that cancer has also recurred elsewhere in the body, the recurrence may be better treated with systemic treatment such as chemotherapy or hormones.

Studies have been done to determine whether chemotherapy added to surgery and/or radiation will cure more women with local relapse than surgery and/or radiation alone. Although these trials have not yet shown a definite benefit of adding chemotherapy, if the woman is young and has not had previous chemotherapy, it may be recommended after the local recurrence has been removed.

Cancer recurrence in the breast after partial mastectomy and radiation

Cancer may recur in the breast after conservative surgery and radiation in approximately 10% of women during the 10 years following treatment. Sometimes, recurrence in the breast can be treated for cure, but this often requires a mastectomy. A recurrence in the breast after a partial mastectomy and radiation has a better prognosis than a local recurrence on the chest wall after a mastectomy, and is often not associated with any other relapse. To detect a small, curable recurrence we recommend physical examinations and mammography every year, starting about six months after the radiation is finished.

The chance of a recurrence after partial mastectomy alone without radiation is higher, but can be treated with a repeat lumpectomy. Radiation at this time is usually advised. However, it is not usually possible to repeat a course of radiation if this was used after the initial surgery.

Treatment of a local recurrence after mastectomy

Recurrence of breast cancer may occur on the chest wall, or in lymph glands in the armpit (axilla), above the collar bone (supraclavicular fossa) or behind the breast bone (internal mammary nodes). If the patient has not previously received radiation then the usual treatment is to remove the recurrence surgically (if it is small and localized) and then give radiation therapy (see Chapter 25). If the recurrence is very extensive, with growth to the bones, muscles or nerves, or cancer recurs within the chest wall and lymph glands after previous radiation therapy, or if recurrence is found at the same time in other organs like the lungs, treatment needs to be individualized. However, in these situations it is usual to use hormones or chemotherapy as the first approach.

CHAPTER FORTY

Treatment of recurrence elsewhere in the body (metastasis)

Why does the cancer recur elsewhere?

CANCER COMES BACK elsewhere in the body (a 'systemic recurrence') because breast cancer cells escaped into the blood stream prior to the first treatment. Although adjuvant chemotherapy and hormone therapy is given to try to destroy these cells, it is not always effective. Cells that are resistant to the drugs are not killed and may divide and grow into detectable cancer metastases. Unfortunately, cancer also recurs in some women who were initially thought to be at low risk of a relapse.

What can I expect if I have a recurrence elsewhere?

The behavior of the returning cancer seems to depend on a number of factors, including:

a) the amount of time passed since the original cancer was diagnosed: the more time in between the better the outcome
b) the type of cancer: the less aggressive, the better
c) the tumor's estrogen receptor status: estrogen receptor-positive tumors respond better to treatment than estrogen receptor-negative tumors

d) the number of tumor sites: the fewer, the better; and
e) the sites of the metastases: for example, bone metastases are often slower growing than liver metastases.

The most important factor, however, is how the cancer responds to therapy. If the cancer responds to one type of treatment, then it is more likely that other treatments will also be effective in controlling it. If the cancer does not shrink in response to any of the usual treatments, the outlook is not as good.

What are the signs of systemic recurrence?

The most common sites for breast cancer spread are the bones, lung, liver and brain. However, other parts of the body can also be affected. When breast cancer spreads, the cells still look and behave like the original breast cancer. Therefore, if a breast cancer spreads to the lung, it is still breast cancer (not lung cancer). This is important because the types of treatment and the chance of success are different for a spreading breast cancer than for a lung cancer.

The symptoms of breast cancer spread depend on the part of the body affected. Cancer in the bones usually causes progressively increasing pain or a spontaneous fracture (a broken bone). In the lungs, it may cause cough or shortness of breath. In the liver it causes loss of appetite, pain in the upper abdomen and sometimes jaundice. If cancer spreads to the brain it may cause headache, numbness or weakness of an arm or leg, loss of balance, confusion or seizures depending on which part of the brain is affected.

This list of potential problems may be frightening, and a woman may find herself constantly checking for new problems. This is quite normal. Many women report being much more aware of their bodies and of having frequent fears of recurrence, especially in the first year or two after treatment. You should feel comfortable enough to ask your doctors about these concerns. The important things to report are persistent changes in your body's function. Symptoms that come and go within 24 hours are not a sign of cancer.

What are the goals of treatment?

The goals of treatment of metastatic breast cancer are to relieve symptoms, maintain quality of life, and prolong survival. The word 'cure' comes up with hopes for a successful treatment of the systemic recurrence. However, disappointment often follows when the physician cannot guarantee or even predict promising results. Many people live with longstanding (chronic) diseases that cannot be cured, such as heart disease, emphysema, diabetes, and arthritis, in which treatment is not curative but is given to avoid severe complications and symptoms. Metastatic breast cancer can be similar to one of these chronic diseases, with a series of treatments given to decrease the symptoms and avoid complications. After a systemic recurrence, breast cancer is usually not curable. However, the length of life can be as much as ten years or more, and it is impossible to accurately predict how long a particular individual may survive.

The treatments

Patients with metastatic breast cancer usually receive a sequence of treatments, including hormones, radiotherapy, chemotherapy, nutritional support, pain management, psychological support, and sometimes surgery. Even after a diagnosis of recurrence is made, the best treatment for a woman with *no symptoms* may be *no treatment* until symptoms occur. This is because a treatment may have side effects that are worse than the disease. Judging whether to give treatment is sometimes a delicate balance. A metastatic tumor may simply be watched for a month or two (if it is not causing problems) to chart how quickly it is growing.

Systemic (whole body) therapy with hormones or chemotherapy should be given if there is widespread symptomatic cancer, if the cancer seems to be growing rapidly, or if there is widespread involvement of organs that is impairing their function.

The type of systemic therapy initially used depends on a number of factors:

a) the type of the original tumor: whether it was estrogen receptor-positive
b) the length of time since the original diagnosis: a long period of time despite an initial estrogen receptor-negative tumor may suggest a hormone-responsive cancer
c) the organs involved: bone metastases may respond better to hormones
d) the severity of the symptoms: with widespread cancer in the lungs the patient cannot wait until the tumor responds to hormone therapy, and
e) the age of the patient: chemotherapy may be too harsh for an elderly woman with other health problems.

When is hormone therapy used?

For most systemic recurrences the first therapy used is hormones. Even if the original cancer was an estrogen receptor-negative tumor, if a few years have passed since that diagnosis, the cancer may respond. However, if the cancer is growing rapidly in vital organs such as the lungs or liver, hormones may not be the best treatment because they often take a couple of months to show an effect, and the cancer may be causing severe problems by then. The therapies with the fewest side effects are used first, followed by ones that are less well tolerated. This approach is used to maintain an optimal quality of life. Unfortunately, even if there is a good response to a particular hormone, the response does not last forever. Other hormone drugs may then be tried until the cancer either no longer responds or is growing rapidly in a vital organ such as the liver or lungs.

Postmenopausal women

For postmenopausal women, tamoxifen is usually the first treatment. If the cancer recurs a few years after adjuvant tamoxifen has been discontinued, the recurrence may respond to another course of this hormone. However, if the cancer recurs very soon after completion of or during the adjuvant treatment, there is less chance of seeing a response to tamoxifen.

Premenopausal women

For premenopausal women the initial hormone treatment can be either tamoxifen or reduction of estrogen by surgical removal of the ovaries or radiation of the ovaries. (Removing the ovaries from postmenopausal women is of no value since they are no longer producing estrogens.) A new medication, Zoladex®, also works by stopping the production of estrogen in the ovaries.

For how long can hormone therapy be used?

Hormone therapy is usually continued until the recurrent cancer no longer responds. Most oncologists try one or two hormones before deciding whether the tumor is responding or not. All hormones act slowly, so the tumor's response can't be assessed before six to twelve weeks, although the patient may begin to feel better before that. Since the hormones are used in order of increasing side effects, many clinics start with tamoxifen, and then follow with aromatase inhibitors (Arimidex® or Femara®), megestrol (Megace®), fluoxymesterone (Halotesin®), or medroxyprogesterone.

When is chemotherapy used?

Chemotherapy is used as the first treatment for a systemic recurrence when the tumor is not likely to respond to hormones. This may include a fast-growing tumor, one that occurs soon after the initial diagnosis, or an estrogen receptor-negative cancer. Chemotherapy is also used to treat cancers that have not responded to a trial of hormone therapy or those which initially responded but are no longer doing so.

How is an appropriate chemotherapy combination chosen?

The choice of drugs to treat the metastatic cancer depends on previous treatment that the woman has had and the amount of time between any adjuvant chemotherapy and the recurrence. Drugs may be given individually or in combinations with other drugs. If a woman has had no previous chemotherapy, the most effective drug combination usually consists of doxorubicin

(Adriamycin®), cyclophosphamide and 5-fluorouracil. If the patient is elderly or has a significant heart problem, doxorubicin is not usually used. If adjuvant chemotherapy was given, but more than a year before the recurrence, the same drugs may be used as before, possibly in a new combination.

There are a number of newer drugs that are also effective in treating recurrent breast cancer. These include, among others, docetaxel (Taxotere®), paclitaxel (Taxol®) and vinorelbine (Navelbine®). As well, there are a number of older drugs that may also be useful, including methotrexate, epirubicin, 5-fluorouracil, mitomycin, mitoxantrone, vinblastine, cisplatin, and thiotepa. The choice of drugs depends on the woman's previous chemotherapy, her general health, the side effects that she and her oncologist are comfortable with, and where and how rapidly her disease is growing.

New drugs are continuously being studied with the hope that they may be more effective in treating breast cancer.

What are the side effects?

The side effects of the chemotherapy depend on which drugs are used and the doses, and vary from one person to another. Docetaxel can commonly cause a decrease in the white blood cell count which can lead to severe infection, so it is important that any fever, chills, cough, pain with urination or other signs of infection be reported immediately. As well, docetaxel can cause hair loss, thin nails and sometimes an accumulation of fluid, resulting in swelling of the legs, arms or abdomen. Paclitaxel causes hair loss, a lowering of the white blood cell count and risk of infection, muscle aches and pains a few days after the chemotherapy infusion, and tingling in the fingers and toes. People can get an allergic reaction to docetaxel or paclitaxel. To avoid this, a steroid (dexamethasone) is given for two to three doses before the chemotherapy and has been shown to decrease the chance of a reaction.

Vinorelbine causes nausea and vomiting, constipation, muscle aches and pains and, occasionally, a burning sensation in the vein after it is given.

Ask your doctor and the oncology nurse to carefully explain the details of the side effects you may expect, as these will depend on which drugs have been ordered for you. As well, make sure to ask whom to call if you have any problems.

For how long is chemotherapy continued?

Chemotherapy may be given for a set number of courses or may be continued for as long as there is evidence of response. If there is a good response to the first course of chemotherapy, a second type of chemotherapy may be tried when the cancer recurs. If the cancer does not respond to two different types of chemotherapy, it may be a very stubborn and resistant cancer. In this situation the oncologist may decide to avoid further chemotherapy if it is causing side effects and not benefitting the patient.

Often, chemotherapy can effectively decrease the symptoms of metastatic cancer, such as the shortness of breath that may occur if the cancer is in the lungs. It can also reduce bone aches, enlarged lymph nodes, tumors of the skin or liver, or tumors in the abdomen. Unfortunately it can rarely overcome the fatigue that is a common complaint of women with recurrent cancer.

Studies are evaluating high-dose chemotherapy and bone marrow transplants as treatments for women with systemic recurrences, but this has not been shown to be a better treatment than standard-dose chemotherapy.

When is radiation used to treat systemic recurrences?

Radiation can be given for recurrent tumors that cause symptoms in a specific area of the body. This includes recurrent tumors in the lymph nodes in the chest that cause shortness of breath, tumors near the esophagus that interfere with swallowing, or tumors in the bones, brain and other structures.

The decision to treat with radiation is based on several factors: the site of the recurrence, the symptoms that may be relieved by the treatment, the symptoms that may be caused by the treatment, and how much radiation the area has received in the past. Organs in the body tolerate radiation differently.

Some areas can only be treated once or can only tolerate low doses of radiation, while other areas can be retreated or given high doses.

Radiation can be given either at the same time as hormones or chemotherapy, or by itself. Radiation can often successfully decrease pain, particularly bone pain. The relief from pain occurs because radiation kills cancer cells, causing tumors to shrink and pressure in the bones to be relieved. The pain relief may be immediate or gradual over a month or so. Bones tolerate higher doses of radiation than many other tissues, so depending on the doses used, a bone can sometimes be treated with radiation more than once.

If the cancer recurs in the chest wall, radiation may be used to treat the recurrence even if there is also evidence of cancer elsewhere in the body. Various types of radiation can be used for recurrences on or under the skin, depending on how deep the metastases are and how much radiation has been given before.

The mainstay of treatment for a cancer that recurs in the brain is radiation treatment of the brain to shrink the cancer. The side effects of the therapy may include fatigue, mild nausea and headaches. Hair loss always occurs when the whole brain is treated with radiation, but it begins to grow back after three or four months.

Can surgery be used to treat systemic recurrences?

Yes, sometimes. If there are bone metastases, surgery may be used to stabilize the bone to avoid fractures, or to mend bones that have already broken. Pins or plates can be used to make the bone more stable and to decrease pain. Occasionally, surgery may be used to remove a lump or recurrence on the skin even when there is evidence of other metastases.

If the woman is in reasonable overall shape and has only one site of metastatic disease, surgery can be used to remove it from the lungs, liver or brain, especially in cases of slow-growing tumors. With breast cancer, however, it is rare to have just a single metastasis, so very few patients are considered for this treatment. Since the cancer cells travel in the blood stream, the surgical removal of a single visible lump will not likely cure the cancer by removing it from that one site.

Tumors may be removed from the brain if they are solitary, easily accessible, or not suitable for radiation. Although this may ease the symptoms, the long-term outlook is not good.

Treatment of fluid accumulation

Recurrent breast cancer can cause excessive fluid to accumulate around the lungs (pleural effusion) due to blockage of normal lymphatic drainage. This can cause shortness of breath or a sharp chest pain that worsens when taking a deep breath. Physical examination and a chest x-ray will diagnose it. It is usually treated with a 'chest tube' to drain the fluid. Once the fluid is gone, a drug (often doxycycline or bleomycin) or talcum powder is put into the pleural space to close it and prevent the fluid from reaccumulating.

Fluid may also accumulate in the abdomen and cause an uncomfortable swelling of the belly. A physician can usually make the diagnosis with a physical examination and confirm it with an ultrasound. If the fluid causes discomfort, temporary relief can be obtained if a catheter is inserted into the abdomen to drain the fluid. However, the fluid usually reaccumulates very quickly unless some other treatment of the cancer is given, such as chemotherapy or hormone treatment.

What can I do for myself?

Nutrition

Good nutrition is very important in maintaining a sense of well-being; studies have not shown that diet alone can treat metastatic cancer. For many women with a recurrence, eating becomes difficult because they are fatigued or nauseated. In this situation, consultation with a nutritionist is important to learn ways to maintain an adequate diet. Chapter 36 discusses some of these issues.

Pain management

Pain may be present during recurrent breast cancer. Although radiation and systemic therapy may provide some relief, the use of regular and adequate medication is important to avoid letting the pain build up. It is important for you to find a drug that you tolerate well. With a physician's guidance you can increase the dose until the pain is relieved.

Many patients are uneasy about taking medications for pain, particularly if they are worried that the pills may be addictive or if they feel that taking medication for pain is a sign of 'giving in.' These thoughts are common. Most people will not become addicted to medications that are given to treat pain, and since being pain-free is essential for a good quality of life, it is not a 'weakness' or a sign of 'giving in' to treat the pain. It is simply allowing you to continue as many activities as possible for as long as possible. Unfortunately, all 'pain killers' have side effects. Narcotic medications (codeine, morphine and others) most commonly cause constipation. This can be avoided by taking stool softeners and adequate dietary fiber and fluids as soon as the narcotic medication is started. Bone pain is sometimes decreased by using biphosphonates (clodrinate, pamidronate, etc.)

Mental well-being

Psychological well-being is also a very important part of the treatment of recurrent disease. Although the support of friends and family is crucial, individual counselling or discussion with a group of women with recurrent cancer may provide another means of support. Relaxation groups, massage therapy or other types of therapy may also help you cope with this new and frightening situation (see Chapter 37). Some research suggests that women who regularly participate in group counselling sessions with other women tend to survive longer. We encourage women to seek out group support therapy.

Palliative care

Palliative care concentrates on relieving the symptoms caused by the cancer rather than treating the cancer itself. Many centers have specialized palliative care teams that provide in-hospital and home care. These teams work cooperatively with the patient and her family to maintain an optimal quality of life while remaining in her home setting for as long as possible. One of the goals is to allow the woman independence, dignity and choices during the difficult final phase of her life. Particular attention is paid to pain relief, nutrition, bowel care, psychological support and family needs.

SECTION FIFTEEN

Special Topics

CHAPTER FORTY-ONE

Breast cancer and pregnancy

THIS CHAPTER ANSWERS three questions:

1. What are my options if I receive a diagnosis of breast cancer while I am pregnant?
2. Does treatment of breast cancer affect my fertility?
3. Can I become pregnant after I have completed treatment for breast cancer?

If breast cancer is diagnosed during pregnancy

The procedure for diagnosing breast cancer is generally the same in the pregnant and the nonpregnant woman. Of course, care is taken to protect the fetus during chest x-rays by providing appropriate shielding. Also, bone scans should not be done since some of the radioactive particles may get into the fetus.

Deciding on a treatment plan

Treatment of breast cancer during pregnancy must be individualized: the woman and her family must be intimately involved in the decision-making. There are a number of special factors to consider, including the stage of the cancer, the type of treatment required, and the gestational age of the fetus.

In general, surgical therapy (mastectomy and axillary dissection) is safe and can proceed. Termination of pregnancy may be discussed. It has not been shown to have any beneficial effect on the cancer, but may allow earlier treatment with chemotherapy and/or radiation if they are required. This is because chemotherapy and radiation can have harmful effects on the fetus, particularly in the first third of pregnancy. In some circumstances mastectomy is appropriate, with adjuvant treatment delayed until after the birth. Occasionally, if the cancer is progressing very rapidly, a small risk of harm to the fetus may be accepted and chemotherapy or radiotherapy may be started, even while the fetus is still growing.

An obstetric evaluation should be done to determine the exact age of the fetus to help decide on the best time to deliver the baby. If an early delivery is an option, it should proceed before the breast cancer treatment starts. A delay in treatment of about four weeks is generally unlikely to affect the mother's chances of being cured, and will allow the baby to mature and have a better chance of being born healthy. The goal of any treatment is to achieve a good result for both the mother and the child. Each woman's situation is different, and requires careful consideration of all these options and in-depth discussion between the patient, her family, obstetrician, oncologist and surgeon to arrive at the best treatment plan.

Myths to dispel about breast cancer and pregnancy

Breast cancer is *not* more aggressive and does not have a worse outcome when it is discovered during pregnancy. Breast cancer does *not* spread to the fetus. Also, abortion of the fetus does not usually improve the outcome or have an effect on the growth of the mother's cancer.

Is fertility affected by breast cancer treatment?

Premenopausal women who receive chemotherapy may have their menstrual periods stop permanently and they may become infertile. This is more likely to occur as a woman gets older and nears the time of her normal menopause. For example, approximately 30% of women younger than 40 years but nearly all women older than 45 years will enter menopause after six months of chemotherapy. Sometimes menstruation returns six months to a year after chemotherapy is completed. However, since many women do remain fertile while receiving chemotherapy it is important to use effective methods of contraception (but not birth control pills) if you are sexually active. Radiation, unless it is directed at the pelvis, will not affect fertility. Tamoxifen (hormone therapy) may cause menstrual irregularities but does not make women infertile. Women must use effective contraception while taking tamoxifen.

Even if your menstrual periods are unaffected, it is recommended that you do not get pregnant until at least six months after completing treatment. Any residual effects of chemotherapy or scattered radiation to the ovaries should have resolved by then.

Pregnancy after breast cancer

Women who get pregnant after having breast cancer have the same long-term outcome as women who have had breast cancer who do not become pregnant. There is no evidence that getting pregnant makes the cancer regrow or spread any more frequently or faster than if the woman does not get pregnant. There is also no increased chance of fetal malformations among babies born to women who have had breast cancer or treatment for breast cancer in the past.

Following radiation therapy of the breast, the normal breast tissue is permanently altered. The normal engorgement in preparation for lactation does not occur, and during lactation very little, if any, milk is produced from the irradiated breast. This means that the breasts may become quite lopsided during pregnancy. However, breastfeeding from the unaffected breast is still possible and is encouraged.

Making the decision about whether to become pregnant

Apart from the biological considerations, a woman and her partner need to consider various social, psychological and economic implications of bearing a child. This is doubly hard when the mother-to-be is uncertain of her future. Often, delaying pregnancy for at least six months or more after breast cancer treatment is completed is a good idea, as it allows the woman's body and mind time to heal. Beyond these considerations there is no medical reason to delay pregnancy beyond six months. However, some doctors recommend a delay of two to five years to have greater confidence that the cancer won't recur.

In the final analysis, the woman, together with her family, needs to weigh the various possibilities, including her age, her risk of cancer recurrence, the desire to have a baby, and her ability to care for the child if cancer recurs. If the woman and her family are counselled well, she can be encouraged to become pregnant if she so wishes.

CHAPTER FORTY-TWO

Familial breast cancer and genetic testing

by Charmaine Kim-Sing, MD

Do my daughters have a higher risk of breast cancer?

THIS IS A FREQUENTLY asked question. At the outset, it is important to say that most daughters will not get breast cancer. However, because your daughters are female this means that they live with at least the 'average' risk of any woman. We also know that breast cancer can be passed on in families (Chapter 4) so the question really becomes, 'How much higher than the normal risk do my daughters face?'

To evaluate your daughter's risk of developing breast cancer several points need to be considered:

- How old were you when you developed breast cancer?
- Did the cancer affect one or both breasts?
- How many of your close relatives have breast cancer?
- How old is your daughter?
- Does your daughter have any other risk factors?

Your age at diagnosis

As women get older, the chance of developing breast cancer increases. This is unrelated to any special inherited tendency (see Chapter 3). Therefore, if the mother develops breast cancer at an older age, for example 75, the daughter's risk is only minimally higher. But if the mother developed cancer when she was 40 years old, it is more likely that something 'genetic' contributed to the cause of the cancer, and the daughter has an approximately four to five times higher than normal risk (see Chapter 4).

Cancer of one or both breasts

If both breasts are affected, the chance of a genetic tendency towards breast cancer is higher. If cancer develops in both breasts in a woman younger than 50 years old, this indicates a very substantially higher risk (five to ten times) in her daughters and also in her sisters. There is also evidence that a strong family history of breast cancer on the father's side can be passed on to a daughter, even though the father does not get breast cancer himself.

Number of family members with breast cancer

If many close blood relatives develop breast cancer (or cancer of the ovary or a type of cancer called 'sarcoma'), it is more likely that some genetic error is being passed within the family. This increases the risk to the daughter of an affected woman.

What does 'higher than normal risk' mean in numbers?

It's easiest to illustrate this with an example. Let's say a 58-year-old postmenopausal woman develops breast cancer in one breast and wonders how high her 30-year-old daughter's risk might be. The only other relative with breast cancer was one of the mother's aunts. This family history increases the daughter's risk by about 2.5 times the average. From Table 1 (p. 20), a typical 30-year-old woman has a 1 in 6,000 risk of getting breast cancer each year (not lifetime risk). If the daughter does not have any other risk factors, her chances are now 2.5 times 1 in 6,000 or approximately 1 in 2,400 per year. Over the next 10 years her risk is approximately 1 in 240 or about 0.4%. This is still not a very great risk and is not a reason to undertake any special treatment. The daughter should be aware of the risk, participate in a program of breast health, and begin screening by mammography about ten years before the age at which her mother developed breast cancer (in this case, an age at which she might be recommended to have screening anyway).

Families with a strong history of breast cancer

Approximately 5% to 10% of breast cancers may be due to an inherited genetic mutation. Two genes have already been identified for breast cancer and are named BRCA1 and BRCA2. The mutations are 'spelling errors' or 'mistakes' on specific chromosomes that have been inherited either from the father or the mother. If a mutation is present there is a high risk of developing cancer. In these families, relatives in three or more generations are often affected.

Genetic testing can be done to determine if you have inherited a mutation. Once the mutation is identified in someone who has already been diagnosed with breast cancer, then the relatives of that person can be tested for that mutation. If you are identified as having the abnormal gene, the lifetime risk of developing breast cancer is 60% to 70% and there is also a higher chance of developing cancer in both breasts. BRCA1 also confers a 45% lifetime risk of ovarian cancer. There is a small increased risk of colon cancer and, for males, prostate cancer. BRCA2 confers an increased risk for both male and female breast cancer.

These cancers tend to occur 5 to 10 years earlier in each generation. If an abnormal gene is identified in family members who have breast cancer, individuals who do not inherit the abnormal gene have the same risk for breast cancer as the general population.

Genetic counseling and testing can estimate individual risk

If there is a very strong family history of breast cancer, an unaffected member of the family may be interested in genetic counseling to assess more accurately her individual risk of developing breast cancer. A strong family history is present when there are three or more cases of breast cancer in direct blood relatives, i.e. mother/daughter, aunt/niece, sister or grandmother, including relatives from the father's side. Certain ethnic groups or geographically defined populations have been found to have a high incidence of particular mutations in BRCA1 or BRCA2. For instance, a wide variety of different mutations in BRCA1 are found in approximately 1 in every 1,000 individuals in the general population, but as many as 1 in every 100 Ashkenazi Jewish women have been shown to have three or four specific mutations. Another example is that one mutation accounts for most of the cases of *inherited* breast cancers in Iceland. These commonly occurring mutations in specific populations are called 'founder mutations.' As more research is done, founder mutations will likely be identified in other ethnic groups or geographic populations.

If you decide to have genetic counseling and testing, you will meet with a medical geneticist and/or genetic counselor who will obtain a detailed family history. Your individual risk for breast cancer can be estimated and you will receive counseling regarding the pros, cons and limitations of genetic testing for the abnormal mutation.

High-risk families: criteria for genetic risk assessment

Genetic risk assessment may be beneficial for an individual who is:
- a woman with breast cancer diagnosed at age 35 or younger OR
- a woman with ovarian cancer diagnosed at age 50 or younger OR
- an Ashkenazi Jewish woman with breast or ovarian cancer diagnosed at any age

OR whose family history includes any TWO of the following:
- breast cancer in two or more closely related family members (parents, siblings, children, grandparents, aunts, uncles)
- cancers at an earlier age than expected in the general population (e.g. breast cancer before menopause)
- multiple primary cancers in different organs in one individual

- cancers associated with known hereditary syndromes (e.g. breast/ovary, colon/uterus).

Before having genetic testing done, however, it is important to have counseling to consider the implications of a positive or negative test, and what actions you might take with such information. Counseling will be provided about the limitations of genetic testing, how the results might affect not only your life but that of your family, and how you might use the test results. If you are interested in genetic counseling, have your doctor call your regional cancer center to find out the best way to make a referral.

Hereditary cancer programs

For women who carry an abnormal mutation for breast cancer such as the BRCA1 or BRCA2 genes, some cancer centres provide a high-risk clinic as part of a hereditary cancer program. In these clinics, women are monitored on a specific surveillance program in which screening and regular physical examinations play an important role in the early detection of cancer. Also, recent studies have shown that there are medications that are capable of preventing breast cancer, e.g. tamoxifen and raloxifene (see p. 29). These medications might be prescribed for carefully assessed, high-risk individuals.

Chapter Forty-Three

Male breast cancer

The statistics

MEN DO HAVE BREAST TISSUE and can develop breast cancer, although it is not common. Breast cancer in a man usually appears as a lump under the nipple. Since men are not aware of their risk, they often ignore a lump for months or even years. By then, the cancer may have extended into the skin of the breast, the muscles beneath it and/or the lymph nodes, similarly to a locally advanced (stage III) cancer in a woman (see Chapter 17).

The diagnostic evaluation of the lump should be the same as for a woman and includes the use of bilateral mammograms and biopsy. The chances of survival and of controlling the cancer parallel that of a woman of the same age and depend on the stage of disease at diagnosis. Approximately 85% of breast cancers in men are estrogen-receptor positive.

Treatment

Treatment involves achieving local control, usually by mastectomy and axillary dissection. Breast conservation is rarely an issue for men. Radiation is added if the margins of excision are close to or involve the cancer or if lymph nodes are involved in the axilla. There have been no scientific studies of adjuvant systemic therapy in men because the number of men with breast cancer is so small. In general, however, the course of breast cancer in men is very similar to that in women. Today, many oncologists recommend adding tamoxifen and/or chemotherapy to the local therapy using the same indications as have been described for a woman of the same age in Chapters 28 and 30.

CHAPTER FORTY-FOUR

Alternative and complementary treatments

What are alternative and complementary treatments?

'ALTERNATIVE' AND 'COMPLEMENTARY treatments' are terms for a large number of health therapies that are sometimes referred to as 'unproven' methods of cancer treatment. These methods are not necessarily seen as alternatives to standard therapy, but may be used alongside (complementary to) standard therapy. Many of these treatments 'work' from the point of view of keeping hope alive and giving a woman a sense of control over her life again.

Alternative therapies are a catch-all category that includes a variety of therapies, from vitamins to diets, from relaxation and therapeutic touch to herbal remedies, from immune stimulants to metabolic therapies. It is not clear that all of these therapies should be lumped into one category, but for the purposes of this chapter it is useful to discuss their similarities.

It is estimated that up to 60% of cancer patients participate in some form of alternative therapy. When vitamins, relaxation methods and visualization are included in this category the number is probably larger.

Why are alternative or complementary treatments described as 'unproven'?

Most alternative remedies are referred to as 'unproven' because they have not been subjected to rigorous scientific testing. Physicians depend on extensive experiments and studies to assess new therapies and evaluate their effectiveness. The value of alternative therapies is often based on individual testimonials that the therapy was beneficial, but this is not very dependable information because the particular circumstances and results cannot be confirmed, nor have the remedies been tested in a larger group of people to see if the results can be produced in a consistent way. This is not to say that the treatments have no validity, but most physicians feel uncomfortable placing their faith in a particular remedy without scientific facts to support its use. As well, without more information, it is impossible to know about potential side effects of such treatments — even herbal methods may have severe side effects. It must be acknowledged, however, that much healing occurs outside the realm of science.

Why do patients use non-traditional treatments?

Many women seek alternative therapy when they feel that their physicians predict only 'doom and gloom.' If the oncologist appears to have little to offer or if standard treatments offer little chance for cure, it is appealing to try something that seems hopeful and positive. As well, many of the practitioners of holistic approaches are very charismatic and optimistic. Who wouldn't seek the reassurance of a practitioner who gives hope rather than one who seems more negative?

Many women also adopt complementary treatments because they feel empowered in choosing and directing their own care. This is a very positive attitude that helps one's psychological health during the ordeal of cancer therapy. This assertiveness shouldn't be restricted to choosing methods of alternative therapy. Each patient should participate in the decisions regarding her conventional treatment: the type of surgery, radiation, chemotherapy and hormones.

Not only does the patient often feel powerless, but so do many friends and family members, who may steer patients towards non-traditional treatments because they want to help. Other patients simply have a general mistrust of the conventional medical establishment.

Alternative treatments often seem less toxic and more natural, with claims of boosting an individual's own immune system to attack the cancer in a natural way. Many patients claim that holistic programs are gentler, less invasive and more individualized.

Types of alternative treatments

The most common alternative cancer therapies can be categorized into the following groups: metabolic therapies, herbal remedies, mega-vitamins, diet therapy, visual imagery and immune therapy. There are also a large number of treatments that cannot be described in detail here, but more complete descriptions are available (see Additional Reading).

Metabolic therapies

The concept of metabolic therapies is that toxins in the body cause and promote cancer, and that certain agents will detoxify the body, including laetrile, iscador (made from mistletoe) and hydrazine. Laetrile was tested in a large study run by the National Cancer Institute in the USA which failed to show that it was beneficial. As well, there have been some laetrile-related deaths, possibly due to the cyanide which is an active ingredient. The other treatments, iscador and hydrazine, have not been studied scientifically so it is difficult to assess their risks or benefits.

Herbal remedies

Herbal remedies have been used by healers for hundreds of years. Some of these remedies have been found to contain active agents that have become modern medicines. These include chemotherapy drugs such as vincristine and vinblastine from the periwinkle plant. Others, however, are considered to have secret, curative properties which remain untested. Comfrey, taheebo tea and Essiac can be included in the latter group. Essiac, which is now sold under a variety of names such as 'Fluressence,' was used initially by a nurse in Ontario to treat cancer in the 1920s. A large number of testimonials claimed that it had curative properties. For years the tea was distributed through the Canadian Health Protection Branch until the product became commercially available. In the 1980s a company did a scientific study of Essiac, but the results have never been published and are not available. Herbal remedies may not be completely safe; comfrey can cause liver damage and other herbs have been reported to be contaminated by dangerous fungi.

Mega-vitamins

Many people support mega-vitamin use. Vitamins are necessary for many of the chemical reactions in the body. It is claimed that high doses of vitamins, particularly vitamin C, can kill cancer cells and heal tissues. Although a normal diet contains adequate amounts of vitamins for usual activities, there may be some benefit from higher doses of some vitamins. Unfortunately, all vitamins can cause severe side effects if the doses are too high, so a vitamin program should be discussed with your doctor.

Diet

'You are what you eat' is a phrase we have all heard. With respect to cancer, diet has been suggested as a cause by some and as a treatment by others. Various diets have been proposed as therapies for cancer. These include macrobiotic diets, vegetarian diets, grape diets, the Mormon diet and many others. However, without there being a simple cause for cancer, it is difficult to imagine that a diet alone can cure all malignancies; on the other hand, dietary changes may be helpful in promoting overall health (see Chapter 36).

Immune therapy

Many treatments can be included in this group. These all depend on the theory that cancer is due to an immune defect, so if the immune system can be strengthened, then the cancer can be controlled. Although some cancers do seem to be directly

---

Open discussion builds trust

Although many patients are hesitant to discuss their interest in alternative methods of cancer treatment, it is important that the physician be informed for the benefit of both the patient and the doctor.

In an open and trusting atmosphere with their doctor, women need to be given the opportunity to explore these treatments. It is also necessary for physicians to explore and learn about these therapies to be able to advise and support their patients. There may be some therapies that are proven effective in some cases, or which lead to new discoveries. Physicians can also learn that some of the appeal of these therapies is the hope and optimism that they provide. Conventional medicine can learn that promoting a positive attitude can help, even in the most trying situations.

Patients who opt for alternative or complementary treatments should not be hesitant to maintain contact with, or return to, their conventional doctors when the time seems right.

---

related to the immune system, others occur without any obvious connection to our immune system, which is a very complex and poorly understood part of our make-up. Researchers and immunologists are struggling to determine what role the immune system has in the treatment of various cancers. At this time, despite years of research, there are many unanswered questions. Vaccines and medications to boost the immune system have validity for some cancers, but there is no evidence that immune stimulation is beneficial against breast cancer.

Visual imagery and other forms of 'mental energy'

The concept of visual imagery is that mental energy can be focused through visualization to destroy cancer cells or stop their growth. Relaxation groups and meditation rely on the premise that a healthy mental attitude can aid healing. As well, other methods such as therapeutic touch, massage therapy and other physical techniques rely on the concept of the connection between mental attitude and physical health. While these therapies have not been proven to act on their own, they promote one's sense of responsibility and control in a way that can act with other healing remedies. The field of neuroendocrinology explores the connection between stress, health and the immune system and may lead to some important discoveries and treatments.

What are the risks of these treatments?

The risks of alternative therapies are related to the lack of scientific testing. We depend on regulations to keep our food safe. We test and categorize which additives are approved, and legally require that they be listed on the box or package to protect us as consumers. None of these safeguards exist for alternative cancer treatments. As well, the costs can be prohibitive. A therapy that promises a 'cure' makes people with cancer susceptible to paying potentially large amounts of money regardless of the lack of firm evidence of benefit.

The practitioners of alternative treatments may be very ethical and well-meaning, but there are no safeguards to protect patients from quacks and crooks that are also in the business. It is important that patients who seek alternative therapies be directed to people with a reputation for honesty and reasonable cost.

Another problem is that if the cancer does not respond to a change in, say, behavior or diet, the patient then feels like a failure. Many people already (mistakenly) feel totally responsible for getting cancer in the first place — due to their diet, or stress in their past. Although accepting responsibility for making treatment choices is worthwhile, blaming oneself can be very damaging.

Finally, some cancers are very treatable and can be cured with standard therapy. Although every patient should have a choice of treatment, there are concerns that when curative treatment is rejected in favor of an alternative therapy, the chance of being cured may be lost because of a delay in initiating the proper anti-cancer treatment.

CHAPTER FORTY-FIVE

Clinical research:
Looking for better answers

Why are clinical studies important?

As MOST WOMEN quickly learn, there are a lot of unanswered questions about breast cancer (and many other diseases). What is/are the cause(s)? Can we prevent it? What new treatment or approach might give better results than we're getting right now? Is there some way of curing breast cancer permanently?

Research studies (also called 'trials') are set up to try to answer these and other questions. It's an ongoing process, with questions constantly being asked, and researchers constantly looking for better ways of treating patients in every area of medicine. Sometimes we even forget that the treatments we're using now for breast cancer (drugs, surgery, radiation) were at one time part of a study in which a group of researchers were trying something new.

What are the steps in testing a new treatment?

All potential treatments go through the same type of rigorous evaluation process that can be illustrated with the example of the testing of a new drug.

292

All new drug treatments begin in the laboratory. If extensive tests in test tubes and mice show that a new drug has potential in treating breast cancer, then it is tested in humans in a preliminary (phase 1) study to check on side effects and to establish a dose for which the side effects are acceptable. Then, the drug is tested in a small group of women to determine its effect in controlling the cancer (phase 2). At this stage the question is, 'Does the drug work at a dose that is safe in humans?' Phase 1 and 2 studies usually involve women with advanced or metastatic breast cancer.

If the results are still promising, the question then arises whether the new drug is better than the 'standard' treatment. To determine this, a third (phase 3) study is done in which women are randomly selected for either the new or old treatment. If it is not known which treatment is superior, it is ethical to compare the treatments in consenting, volunteer women.

Scientific studies such as these must follow rigid statistical rules to confirm that the information gained is reliable and repeatable. It is also important to realize that patients must give their consent before they are included in any study.

What should I do if I'm asked to be part of a study?

Participation in any study is strictly voluntary. It is important for any patient enrolling in a study to understand why it is being set up, what is already known of the treatment's side effects and benefits and what the alternatives are. Many phase 2 and 3 trials use drugs that have been studied already, so there may be considerable information available on the treatment. On the other hand, it is important to understand that the primary aim of a phase 1 trial is to define the side effects.

Before any study is done, hospital ethics committees evaluate each study to ensure that the rights of the patients are protected and that the study is ethical in its design and implementation. These ethics committees always include members of the lay public. An informed consent must be obtained from each patient before enrolment in the study. The researcher must carefully discuss the study with each potential participant, explaining the reasons for it, the risks and benefits, and other options the patient has in terms of treatment. The patient should not sign unless she has had all her questions answered thoroughly.

Ultimately, each woman must feel free to decide what is in her best interests, and must be comfortable in choosing to be a part of a study. Also, she must understand that her standard of care will not change if she subsequently decides to withdraw from it. It is through the commitment of thousands of women participating in clinical research that many advances have been made in the treatment of breast cancer.

CHAPTER FORTY-SIX

New directions in breast cancer therapy

RESEARCHERS ARE CONTINUALLY trying to improve our methods of diagnosing and treating breast cancer. We are learning more about how a cancer cell grows, what genetic information is important, and how we can develop drugs or therapies to stop the growth of cancer cells. Both the ways in which cells grow and die may be abnormal in a cancer cell.

Markers of cell growth

From new laboratory tests we are recognizing that not all breast cancer cells are alike. These differences may be the key factor in whether a cell travels elsewhere in the body and whether a cancer will respond to a specific drug or not. Many new 'markers' of cell growth are in the testing phase. Tests are being done to discover why some cells are resistant to our therapies and why others respond. From this information, drugs are being tested which increase the sensitivity of cells to chemotherapy and radiation. Some of these drugs act on the cell cover or membrane. Others change the amount of oxygen in the cancer, as this has been shown to be an important variable in many tumors.

Can the spread of cancer be detected?

Positron emission tomography (PET) scanners are one of the new machines that may help us diagnose the spread of cancer more efficiently. Using radioactive 'tags' on cells we may soon be able to track cells throughout the body and make treatment plans according to the results. As well, researchers are using new methods to study the bone marrow of women at the time of the diagnosis of breast cancer to see if information from the bone marrow can help us determine if cancer cells have spread. These types of studies may be important in helping to give specific therapies to women who are at risk of recurrence and to avoid chemotherapy in those women who have no evidence of meta-static disease.

Antibody studies

Cancers may have specific proteins on the outer coats or membranes of their cells. Many of these proteins have been identified, and tests are now being done to see if we can create new proteins (antibodies) that will attach to the cell-membrane proteins (antigens) and stop the cell from growing and dividing. Her2Neu is a cell growth promoter protein (also known as c-erb-B2) that occurs in 20% to 30% of breast cancers. Tests of an antibody to Her2Neu have been done and suggest that there may be a role for developing this technology further. Other proteins are also being studied. The challenge will be to find out which proteins need to be blocked in which cancers.

Angiogenesis

As a cancer grows, new blood vessels are formed to bring the necessary oxygen and nutrients to the cells. This is called 'angio-genesis.' Researchers hypothesize that if angiogenesis could be blocked, cancers may both shrink and be unable to metastasize or travel to other parts of the body. Natural products and syn-thetic drugs including thalidomide, shark cartilage and its com-ponents, TNP 470, endostatin and a number of other new products are being tested in the laboratory and in clinical trials. There is the danger that these drugs may disrupt other areas of the body or even cause bleeding. Therefore, information about the safety of these drugs is needed. As well, we do not yet know how effective these drugs will be or when they should be started, i.e. in very early cancer or in more advanced disease.

Antisense therapy

Cells grow due to proteins that are made under the strict directions of the DNA in the cell. The DNA has a specific code, i.e. a 'sense' code. If a new code is introduced into the cell in a short piece of DNA-like material known as 'antisense,' the DNA can be interrupted or confused. This stops the formation of the protein. It is theorized that by stopping the protein, we can stop the growth of the cancer cell. It has been difficult to develop 'antisense' drugs for a number of reasons. The cancer grows due to a large number of proteins so it is not clear whether we can just block one protein. We also need to know which protein is necessary for which cancer. As well, the 'antisense' must get into the cell without first being destroyed in the blood system. Many of these obstacles have been overcome with sophisticated technology, and clinical trials using 'antisense' agents (some also known as oligonucleotides) have begun.

Enzymes

A cell grows by a set of well-defined steps, similar to those in a recipe. At each step, an enzyme, similar to baking powder in a cake recipe, may be required to activate the next step. Understanding these pathways has provided us with new ways to stop the cancer cell growing. Laboratory research is concentrating effort on developing drugs which stop specific enzymes from working. 'Tyrosine kinase' inhibitors are one group of drugs. However, getting these drugs to the cell and avoiding complications in other parts of the body are the challenges to be worked out.

Gene therapy

Gene therapy is a catch-all phrase for a number of types of treatment. The goal is to find the gene which is causing the cancer cell to grow, and to stop it by blocking the enzymes, stopping the DNA, or introducing a new gene into the cell to confuse it. Breast cancer cells are very complicated. No one gene has been identified that is common to all cancers which could be interrupted successfully. But research in the hereditary forms of breast cancer may provide us with more information about how the breast cancer cells grow, and may be able to be help identify new genes that are important in the large proportion of breast cancers that are not due to an inherited gene. As well, a number of studies in other kinds of cancers using this technology may help advance our understanding of breast cancer genetics.

Cancer vaccines

If the body can defend itself against infections, what about the natural defenses against cancer? With infections, we vaccinate the body to stimulate the immune system so we can defend ourselves against the particular bacteria or virus. Similarly, if we can vaccinate with a cancer cell then we may be able to improve the workings of the immune system and the body will be able to rid itself of the cancer. At this time, however, there is no solid evidence that breast cancer is an immune disease. Nor has a specific part of the immune system been found to be deficient in women with breast cancer. However, studies are being done with cancer vaccines in a number of malignancies to see if we can stimulate the body to fight the cancer and control its growth.

The future

There are numerous other areas of study, such as using natural products, finding new chemotherapy drugs, developing specific chemicals by computer technology, and combining chemotherapy with drugs that reverse cell resistance or that simulate the oxygen content of the cell. The future is exciting.

There is the promise of more effective therapies as we target breast cancer more directly using our greater understanding of how cancer cells grow.

CHAPTER FORTY-SEVEN

Awareness and advocacy

by Judith Caldwell, President,
Canadian Breast Cancer Foundation, BC Chapter

I am only one; but still I am one. I cannot do everything; but I can still do something. I will not refuse to do something I can do.

— *Helen Keller*

IN THE LATE 50S, when I was in high school, my friend Cathy's mom developed breast cancer and had radical surgery. We whispered about 'it' behind Cathy's back, but never asked her how everything was at home. We weren't heartless, only young, frightened, embarrassed and unable to find the right words. Perhaps we thought that if we denied that the life of one of our favorite moms was being threatened, that breast cancer would go away and leave us, and our own moms, unscathed.

Decades later, with five years of survival under my belt, I know that silence and denial kill. Our job as advocates is to break the silence and focus an uncompromising light on all the issues surrounding breast cancer.

The effects of this disease can be devastating. While each of us experiences breast cancer differently, most of us ride a roller coaster of overwhelming anxiety, grief, sadness, anger, frustration, hope, denial, black humor… and the fear of a truncated future. On our bodies, there's an indelible physical reminder that our lives have been put in peril, and that breast cancer may return to threaten our lives once again, and perhaps kill us. Advocacy offers a means to channel our energies and to do something positive about a situation over which we still have no means of prevention and precious little control. It's a way to save lives and to forge purpose out of apparent chaos.

Most of us who develop breast cancer are taken by surprise, with no family history or obvious risk factors. We face an instant medical crash course in learning just enough about the disease to make critical treatment choices. Usually, it's not until the immediate crises of diagnosis and treatment decisions have passed that an awareness of the staggering scope of breast cancer emerges. Once the huge numbers of others affected become apparent, a 'Why me?' cry turns into 'Why not me?'

Breast cancer has been around for centuries. So why does it remain a hot, public topic? Is it because our aging population, with active and educated women, is edging into the most susceptible age brackets? Is it because sexual issues are more in the open? Is it because of the growing public awareness of the still sorry amount of funding directed to breast cancer research and education? Is it because advocacy groups have finally emerged, frustrated that other diseases are receiving adequate funding? Is it due to the pointed questions about why there hasn't been more progress in finding preventive strategies and cures, even though the media tout cancer cure 'breakthroughs' on a regular basis?

Advocacy means cornering our politicians who are responsible for allocating money for health issues, and demanding to know how much money has been targeted for breast cancer, and how it is being spent. We have as much right to solid, continued funding as any other widespread, life-threatening disease.

With breast cancer we confront the uncomfortable issue of breasts and the values of femininity, sexuality and nurturing that we have placed upon them. We relish memories of babies nursing at our breasts, a lover's caress and holding those we cherish in a soft embrace. On every newsstand, in every movie and TV show, we are swamped with images exploiting cleavage, with never-ending expectations of how a woman must look to be womanly. The public needs to know that treating breast cancer is about saving life, and that even with changed bodies, life, love, sex and femininity carry on. Indeed, a re-evaluation of priorities and values in the shadow of breast cancer may yield a more conscious appreciation of life.

Raising money is only part of the story of advocacy, however. It is also our job to inform women of the realities of breast cancer and to encourage them to take realistic care of themselves. It is true that thousands of Canadian women have had their futures stolen and die prematurely every year of the disease. It is also true that from 150,000 to 200,000 Canadian women are living with a previous diagnosis of breast cancer.

Across Canada, diagnostic opportunities are unequal, and what is available is not being utilized to the fullest extent. It is tragic that too many women in their most vulnerable years, 50 and over, are not yet using the mammographic screening program available to them. Although the age for beginning screening remains controversial, and it's not yet the 100% perfect early diagnostic solution, I am grateful, as are so many other women, that my tumor was found earlier than it would otherwise have been without this technology. Without it, my tumor would have remained an undetected time bomb in my body for months or years, and I would likely have been faced with much more difficult treatment. Advocacy means taking as much reasonable responsibility for your own health as possible.

Across Canada, information is not easily available for smaller cultural and language groups. Not all women understand how to perform breast self-examination. Not all women know that, if they are diagnosed, there are treatment options and that the earlier the diagnosis, the better the options will be. Not all women realize that their doctors are here to serve them and that they have rights to full information, second opinions and choices. Not all families know that genetic screening clinics are available to give excellent information on the potential susceptibility of women whose families include generations of women who were previously affected by the disease. Our moral support and willingness to accompany others through the maze of new, complex information and difficult choices is also advocacy.

The basic tools of advocacy are information, facts, figures, and a clear understanding of the social and financial impact of the disease. However, breast cancer cannot be 'sold' on finances and numbers alone. The personal is political, and stories of women and families facing breast cancer must be told. The pain of lost battles must be made real and the hope that comes from the lives of long-time survivors spread. As advocates, we must recognize that influence is created and decisions are based on gut reactions as well as logic.

So, what can only one person do?

- **Educate yourself** before you do anything. Learn as much as you can about the disease and the issues that interest you. For example, if funding is your concern, find out how funds are being spent by reading annual general reports of groups raising money. Apply to be part of grant allocation committees.
- **Focus.** Advocacy comes in many forms: support groups, fund-raising, education, concerns about genetic testing or political lobbying. Be bold in asking people with the skills you need to work with you.
- **Find others.** Place an ad in the local newspaper asking for others interested in the issue to contact you. Host a meeting. Many an influential group has first started around a kitchen table.
- **Network strategically.** Consider joining other breast cancer groups locally, provincially, nationally and internationally.
- **Speak out** courageously in public, especially at election time.

The job of finding the cause(s) and ways to prevent breast cancer is a team effort, resembling a marathon more than a sprint. Researchers are people with families and financial obligations like the rest of us. Today, only a few can afford to turn their attention to breast cancer at the current funding levels. We need to attract more money and convince our governments and corporations to set priorities. What could possibly be more important than using corporate donations and tax dollars to save bodies and lives?

Based on the years of basic research that have been done until now, I believe there is realistic hope for dramatic progress within the next decade. With today's knowledge, Cathy's mom would have had a far better chance of being diagnosed earlier, of receiving far less radical treatment, and of living to see her daughter's children.

I know in my bones that one person speaking out can have an impact. Two people determined to bring breast cancer issues forward can move small mountains, and a group of people passionate about making a difference and clear in their goals can mobilize an entire community, indeed, an entire country.

Each of us is only one, but we can still do something.

Glossary

Adjuvant therapy Treatment that is given in addition to the initial surgery (that removes all visible evidence of breast cancer) to help prevent the cancer from recurring. Often called 'insurance' against recurrence of cancer.

Androgen Male hormone that may be used as a drug to treat breast cancer.

Atypical cells Cells that appear abnormal but not cancerous when viewed under the microscope.

Axilla The underarm area between the armpit and the collarbone.

Benign tumor A tumor that is not cancerous.

Biopsy The surgical procedure in which a small piece of tissue is removed to be studied under the microscope to help make a diagnosis.

Breast implant A round or tear drop-shaped sac filled with salt water that is placed under the skin and muscle of the chest wall after mastectomy to recreate a breast shape or improve the shape of an existing breast.

Breast prosthesis An artificial breast form that can be worn externally to replace the breast shape after a mastectomy.

Breast reconstruction Surgical procedures (several types) that recreate a breast shape or nipple after a mastectomy. This may involve insertion of a breast implant or creation of a breast shape from other body tissues.

Calcifications Tiny deposits of calcium that may signify cancer and can be seen on a mammogram.

Carcinoma Another word for cancer.

Cancer The abnormal and uncontrolled growth of cells that may invade and destroy surrounding tissues.

Chemotherapy Treatment for cancer involving the use of drugs.

Clinical trial A carefully designed scientific experiment for testing a new therapy or treatment approach.

Cyst A non-cancerous sac filled with fluid.

Dissection Surgical cutting open of any part of the body.

Edema Swelling of body tissue due to accumulation of fluid. May occur in the arm or breast after removal of lymph nodes during treatment for breast cancer.

Estrogen A sex hormone that is responsible for the development of female characteristics such as breasts and broadening of hips. It also has a key role in the menstrual cycle and pregnancy and stimulates the growth of some breast cancers.

Estrogen receptor A protein in the cancer cell that binds to the hormone estrogen. A cancer cell that is estrogen receptor-rich (or positive) is usually sensitive to hormones.

Fine needle aspiration A biopsy technique in which a thin needle is inserted into the body and a few cells or some fluid is removed for diagnosis.

Fine wire localization A technique to direct a surgical biopsy to an area of the breast which is abnormal on a mammogram but which cannot be felt. A thin wire is placed into the breast under mammographic control to guide the surgeon to the correct part of the breast to be removed.

Hormone therapy Treatment for breast cancer that involves altering the hormone levels in the body. This may involve removing the ovaries or the use of specific drugs.

Hormones Chemicals produced by specific parts of the body (glands) that travel through the blood stream to another location in the body where they cause a change in a structure or function (e.g. estrogen in young women is produced in the ovaries and causes the breasts to develop).

Hyperplasia Cells that divide and accumulate in excessive numbers but are not yet cancerous.

In situ breast cancer Cancer growing within the milk ducts or milk glands of the breast.

Invasive cancer Cancer that has spread from its original location into adjacent tissues or organs.

Lobules (lobular) The milk glands in the breast.

Lumpectomy A surgical procedure in which the tumor and a small margin of surrounding normal breast tissue is removed. Other terms include partial mastectomy, segmental mastectomy, wide excision and breast conservation.

Lymph nodes Small lima bean-shaped structures grouped at various locations along the lymph system in the body (e.g. armpits, neck, groin). They act as the main 'filters' to defend against infections and may be a location to where cancer spreads. Lymph nodes under the arm are frequently removed as part of breast cancer surgery.

Lymphatic system The network of vessels throughout the body that carries lymph fluid to and from all the tissues of the body. Its main function is to fight off infection.

Lymphedema *See* **Edema.**

Malignant tumor A tumor that is harmful because it grows out of control and invades and destroys surrounding tissues.

Mammogram An x-ray of the breast.

Mastectomy The surgical procedure in which the whole breast is removed. Partial mastectomy See Lumpectomy.

Menopause The time of life when a woman's monthly periods stop because her ovaries have stopped making estrogen.

Metastasis The spread of a cancer from one part of the body to another.

Microcalcifications Very tiny calcifications.

Necrosis The death of cells in some part of the body's tissue.

Oncologist A doctor who specializes in the treatment of cancer.

Palpation Examination with the hands; to feel.

Pathologist A doctor who specializes in the structure and function of cells and tissues of the body, and who studies how the various changes relate to specific diseases.

Primary cancer The cancer in the original location where it was first detected.

Progesterone A female sex hormone involved in a number of functions, including the menstrual cycle and pregnancy.

Prognosis An estimate of the expected course of the disease.

Prophylactic A preventive treatment which can involve any type of therapy, e.g. drugs, surgery, radiation.

Prosthesis An artificial device that is attached to the body to substitute for a part of the body that is missing.

Radiotherapy (radiation therapy) The use of high-energy x-rays for the treatment of cancer.

Recurrence The reappearance of cancer following a period of time when there was no evidence of disease. The recurrence may be either at the original site (a local recurrence), in the adjacent lymph nodes (a regional recurrence) or elsewhere in the body (a systemic or distant recurrence).

Risk factor Something that increases your chances of getting a disease, either acquired from the environment, or inherited.

Sarcoma A type of cancer arising from the connecting tissues (muscles, bones, nerves, etc).

Screening Tests done on a person who is feeling well, with no symptoms, to detect evidence of unsuspected disease.

Secondary cancer A cancer that has spread to another site. Also called 'metastatic cancer.'

Staging A procedure involving a variety of tests to establish the extent of the cancer at the time of diagnosis.

Subcutaneous The area underneath the skin.

Sutures Stitches used to close up a surgical wound.

Systemic Affecting the body in general rather than one specific part.

Tamoxifen A drug widely used to treat breast cancer metastases and help prevent the recurrence of breast cancer. It is an anti-estrogen drug since its main action is to block the growth-stimulating effects of estrogen on cancer cells. It is a common form of 'hormone therapy.'

Tumor Abnormal growth of tissue. Can be cancerous (malignant) or noncancerous (benign).

White blood cells Cells in the blood stream that detect and fight infection, 'foreign' material and abnormal cells.

Additional Reading

Healthy eating

Anne Lindsay's light kitchen. Anne Lindsay. MacMillan Canada, Toronto, 1994.

Cancer recovery eating plan: the right foods to help fuel your recovery. Daniel Nixon and Jane Zanca. Random House, Toronto, 1996.

Cancer survivor's nutrition and health guide: eating well and getting better during and after cancer treatment. G. Spiller and B. Bruce. Prima Publishing, 1997.

Nutrition guide for women with breast cancer (booklet). Shirley Hobenshield and Louise Bell. Canadian Cancer Society, Toronto, 1997.

Recipes for health. Cancer: over 100 recipes for coping with cancer during and after treatment. Claire Shaw and Maureen Hunter. Thorsons Publishing Group, San Francisco, 1995.

Smart cooking: quick and tasty recipes for healthy living. Anne Lindsay. MacMillan Publishing, Toronto, 1996.

Complementary and alternative therapy

A guide to unconventional cancer therapies. Ontario Breast Cancer Information Project, Toronto, 1994.

Choices in healing: integrating the best of conventional and complementary approaches to cancer. Michael Lerner. MIT Press, Cambridge, 1994.

Coping/relaxation: Books

Affirmations, meditations and encouragements for women living with breast cancer. Linda Dackman. Harper Collins, New York, 1993.

Cancercervive. Susan Nessin and Joyce Ellis. Houghton Mifflin Co., Boston, 1991.

Dancing in limbo. Glenna Halvorson-Boyd and Lisa Hunter. San Francisco, Jossey-Bass, 1995.

Hands on help: a manual for breast cancer self-help and mutual support groups. Burlington Breast Cancer Support Services, Inc., Burlington, Ontario, 1996.

Helping your mate face breast cancer: tips for becoming an effective support partner. Judy Kneece. Columbia, South Carolina, EduCare Publishing, 1995.

Living beyond limits: new hope and help for facing life-threatening cancer. David Spiegel. Times Books, New York, 1993.

Minding the body, mending the mind. Joan Borysenko. Bantam Books, New York, 1988.

Spinning straw into gold. Ronnie Kaye. Simon and Shuster, New York, 1991.

Man's search for meaning, 4th edition. Viktor Frankl. Boston: Beacon Press, 1994.

Coping/relaxation: Audio and videotapes

Cancer and the whole person (audiotape). Lee Pulos. Hypnosis Development Programs Ltd., 1993.

Healing journey (audiotape). Emmett Miller. Source Cassette Learning Systems, Inc., 1979.

Letting go of stress (audiotape). Emmett Miller. Source Cassette Learning Systems, Inc., 1980.

Significant journey: breast cancer survivors and the men who love them (videotape). American Cancer Society. Minnesota Division. Minneapolis, MN, 1992.

Time in audiotape series 1-7. Lis Smith. Vancouver, B.C., BC Cancer Agency Patient & Family Counselling, 1987-94.

Personal stories: Books/videotapes

A Safe place: A journal for women with breast cancer. Jennifer Pike. Raincoast Books, 1997.

Deep down inside: Ann Jillian talks about the emotional side to cancer (videotape). Ann Jillian. Columbus, Ohio, Adria Laboratories, Inc., 1986.

Holding tight, letting go: living with metastatic breast cancer. Musa Myer. O'Reilly & Associates, Sebastopol, 1997.

Love, Judy: letters of hope and healing for women with breast cancer. Judy Hart. Conari Press, Berkely, Ca, 1993.

My breast. Joyce Wadler. Pocket Books, New York, 1992.

Picasso's woman. Rosalind McPhie. Douglas and McIntyre, Toronto, 1994.

That other place. Penelope Williams. Dundurn Press, Toronto, 1993.

Talking to children: Books/booklets/videotapes

C-word: teenagers and their families living with cancer. Elena Dorfman. NewSage Press, Portland, OR, 1995.

Helping children understand: a guide for a parent with cancer (booklet). American Cancer Society. Minnesota, 1986.

How to help children through a parent's serious illness. Kathleen McCue and Ron Bonn. St. Marin's Press, New York, 1994.

It helps to have friends when mom or dad has cancer. American Cancer Society. Minnesota, 1987.

Mommy's in the hospital again. Carolyn Stearns Parkinson and Elaine Verstraete. Solace Publishing, Inc., Folsom, Ca, 1994.

My mom has breast cancer: a guide for families (videotape). Kidscope, Inc. Atlanta, Ga., 1996.

My mommy has cancer. Carolyn Stearns Parkinson and Elaine Verstraete. Rochester, N.Y., Solace Publishing, 1991.

Talking about your cancer: a parent's guide to helping children cope (videotape). Fox Chase Cancer Center. Philadelphia, 1996.

Vanishing cookies: doing OK when a parent has cancer. Michelle Goodman and Vladyana Krykorka. Benjamin Institute for Community Education and Referral, Downsview, Ontario, 1990.

General Information

Abreast in the nineties (quarterly newsletter). (BC & Yukon Breast Cancer Information Project). Vancouver. (Contact: (604)-872-4400, local 294)

Breast cancer: questions you might want to ask (booklet). Atlantic Breast Cancer Information Project. Canadian Cancer Society, Toronto, 1997.

Dr. Susan Love's breast book. Susan Love and Karen Lindsey. Don Mills, Ontario, Addison-Wesley Publishing, Inc., 1995.

Patient no more: the politics of breast cancer. Sharon Batt. Gynergy Books, 1994.

Recovering from breast surgery: exercises to strengthen your body and relieve pain. Diana Stumm. Hunter House, 1995.

More detailed medical information

Clinical practice guidelines for the care and treatment of breast cancer. A consensus document. The Steering Committee on Clinical Practice Guidelines for the Care and Treatment of Breast Cancer. M. McGregor, editor. Supplement to the *Canadian Medical Association Journal* 1998;158(3 Suppl).

Diseases of the breast (textbook). Jay Harris, Marc Lippman, Monica Morrow, Samuel Hellman. Lippincott-Raven, Philidelphia, 1996.

On the Internet

A breast cancer open discussion forum:
listserv@*morgan.ucs.mun.ca*
write: subscribe breast-cancer (add your name)
An extensive list of breast cancer resources:
http://darkwing.uoregon.edu/~jbonine/bc_sources.html
Breast cancer treatment guidelines and information
for providers and consumers: http://www.bccancer.bc.ca
Canadian Breast Cancer Network: http://www.cbcn.ca
Canadian Cancer Society: http://www.bc.cancer.ca/ccs/
Canadian clinical practice guidelines for the care
and treatment of breast cancer: http://www.cma.ca
NIH Internet site (BIC Breast Cancer Information Core):
http://www.nhgri.nih.gov/Intramural_research/Lab_transfer/Bic/
resources.html
PDQ treatment statements for breast cancer
from USA-National Cancer Institute:
http://www.meb.uni-bonn.de/cancernet/200013.html

Index